GASTRIC SLEEVE COOKBOOK

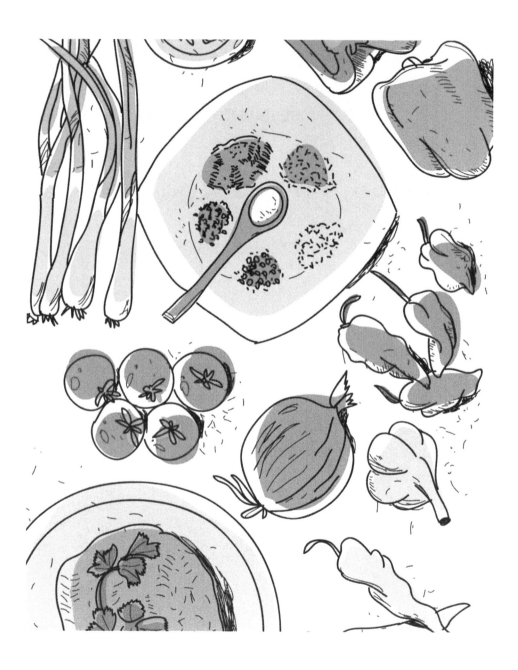

Gastric

SLEEVE

Cookbook

Top 100 Recipes for Every Stage of Bariatric Surgery Recovery

Shannon Henderson

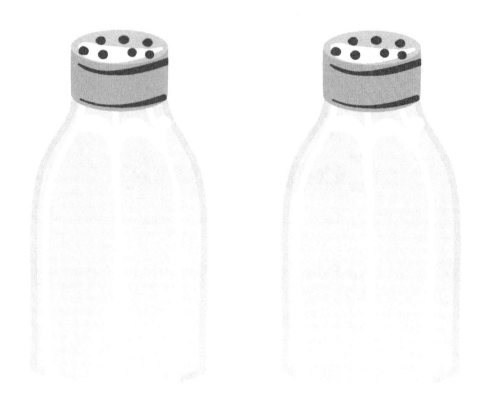

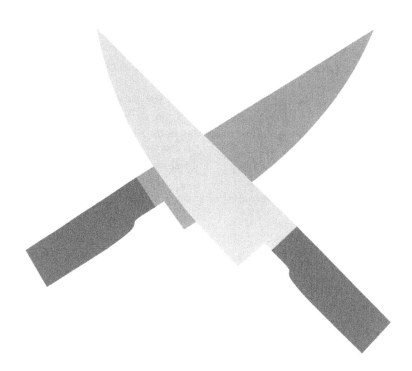

CONTENTS

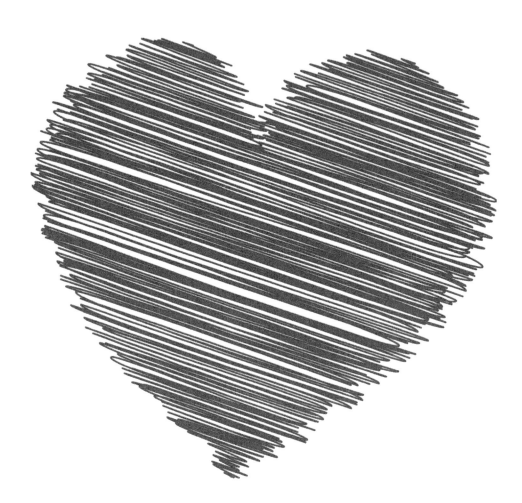

LIFE AFTER WEIGHT LOSS SURGERY

For many years, I struggled with my weight. No matter what I did or changed about my life, I just couldn't lose enough weight. I reached the point where bariatric (weight-loss) surgery became a good option. My surgeon walked me through all the aspects and by following the prep appropriately, my surgery went well.

After gastric sleeve surgery, my diet and how I approached food changed completely. It was challenging at first, especially during recovery, because I needed to weigh my food, count macronutrients, and monitor my nutritional intake. However, it was all necessary in order to heal properly. I knew beforehand that the surgery wouldn't be a magic solution to weight loss, but there are things I didn't know that I wish I had. It would have saved me some discomfort and allowed me to better prepare for challenges that came up. This book collects all that information into one place, so you have a resource you can turn to at any point during your recovery.

We'll go over the different types of weight-loss surgery, why gastric sleeve is a great option, and the possible complications and risks. Once you've had the surgery, you'll enter four phases of recovery where you'll go from drinking only clear liquids, to liquids with protein, to pureed foods, and then introducing solid foods again. The recipe portion of this book will give you ideas on what to eat during these four phases.

Getting enough protein is critical before and after the surgery, so we'll go over different protein shake, water, and bar options. Other types of nutrition like iron and vitamin B12 will also be important, so you'll learn about vitamins and supplements. Long-term weight loss is the ultimate goal of gastric sleeve surgery, so the last part in the introduction gives you ten tips that keep you on track.

Good health is about maintenance and consistency. A gastric sleeve surgery sets you on the right path, but it's all the decisions afterward that really make the difference. I know that being prepared with the information and recipes in this book will help you make the right decisions.

Yours in lasting health and wellness.

Shannon Henderson

INTRODUCTION

Weight-loss surgery, known officially as bariatric surgery, is often necessary if a person is severely obese. It restricts the size of the stomach, so the person can't overeat. This helps significantly with rapid weight loss. It is not a "short cut," however, because the person still needs to eat a healthy diet and exercise, especially if they want to keep excess weight off in the long-term.

Gastric sleeve surgery is one type of weight-loss surgery and quickly becoming the most popular. Around ¾ of the stomach is removed, while the rest of it is joined together to form a sleeve. It is a relatively simple surgery compared to gastric bypass, another common surgery, and requires less maintenance.

In this introduction, you'll learn more about gastric sleeve surgery, including its benefits, risks, and how to prepare for surgery day. You'll also learn how your diet changes following the procedure. It is divided into 4 phases. Along with different eating habits, you'll also be taking vitamins and supplements. Once your recovery is done, you won't go back to your old way of eating. We will go over what successful patients do to stay at a healthy weight.

I. WHAT IS GASTRIC SLEEVE SURGERY?

Also known as a sleeve gastrectomy or vertical sleeve gastrectomy, this surgery was originally just a component of another bariatric procedure. It proved so successful, however, that surgeons expanded their knowledge of it so it could be performed by itself. In North America and Asia, gastric sleeve surgery is the fastest growing weight-loss surgery.

How does the surgery work? It's short at just around an hour. The surgeon makes small cuts in your body to insert a tool called a laparoscope. This sends pictures to a monitor, so the surgeon can see inside you. Using other instruments, the stomach is stapled, removing ¾ of it. The surgeon then joins the rest of it together to make the "sleeve." Your stomach is now just about 1/10 of its original size, so you can't overeat. An added bonus: the part of your stomach that produces an appetite-boosting hormone is removed during the procedure. Hospital time following the surgery is usually two to three days.

OTHER TYPES OF BARIATRIC SURGERY

There are three other types of bariatric/weight-loss surgery that surgeons perform: gastric bypass, a lap-band, and a biliopancreatic diversion with duodenal switch.

Gastric bypass

Gastric bypass is when a surgeon uses staples to divide up the stomach into two parts: one small and one larger. The top part, the pouch, is now your main stomach. Being so much smaller than your original stomach, it holds much less food. The surgeon then connects a small part of your small intestine to the pouch, so food can travel through the body as normal, though now you absorb less calories.

Lap band

The lap-band surgery, known officially as a laparoscopic adjustable gastric band, is when a surgeon puts an inflatable silicone device around the top part of your stomach. This creates a small pouch with a narrow opening to the remaining stomach. You'll feel fuller faster since the band restricts the amount of food your stomach holds.

Benefits to a lap band include no reduction of nutrition absorption, no stomach cutting, and the ability to adjust the band without more surgery. As for risks, internal bleeding, infections, band slippage, stomach pain, and so on have been reported.

Biliopancreatic diversion with duodenal switch

This surgery's name is a mouthful (no pun intended), and requires the removal of a large part (around 70%) of the stomach. The surgeon leaves behind the valve that sends food into the small intestine and the first part of the SI, which is called the duodenum. The "switch" occurs when the doctor separates the middle part of the intestine and attaches the last part to the duodenum.

The separated part of the intestine is then reattached to the intestine *end* to let bile and pancreatic digestive fluids through. The goal of this surgery is to shorten the time the body has to absorb food calories. Patients who get this surgery absorb just 20% of the fat they eat, leading to weight loss. Malnutrition and vitamin/mineral deficiency can also occur, however.

> **There are four types of weight-loss surgeries: gastric sleeve, gastric bypass, lap band, and duodenal switch. Gastric sleeve surgeries take about 1 hour, during which the surgeon removes 75% of the stomach and connects the rest of it to form a sleeve.**

BENEFITS OF A GASTRIC SLEEVE

You know the main types of weight-loss surgery, but why are people choosing a gastric sleeve so often? There are a number of reasons:

Addresses a key element of obesity: appetite

Gastric sleeve is the only surgery that can actually reduce the patient's appetite. This is because the part of the stomach that produces most of the hormone ghrelin, an appetite-creator, is removed. You won't feel the need to eat as often as you did before.

Less complicated than the other types of surgery

Gastric bypass is a complex surgery and takes an average of 4 hours to perform. There is a shorter variation of a gastric bypass surgery, but it's considered very difficult. The duodenal switch surgery is the most complicated because it involves a lot of rearranging. Since it's done in two parts, it can take up to three hours. Lap-band surgery is relatively short at one to two hours and isn't complicated for experienced doctors, but the gastric sleeve surgery only takes an hour and is considered the least challenging.

Doesn't trigger dumping syndrome

When you get parts of your stomach removed, dumping syndrome often results. This happens when sugar moves from your stomach to your small bowel too quickly. You will experience cramps, diarrhea, vomiting, dizziness, and other symptoms 10-30 minutes after eating. Dumping syndrome is especially common after eating meals high in sucrose or fructose. Gastric sleeve patients rarely get this, while it's commonly-associated with gastric bypass surgery.

Results in significant weight loss

Following gastric sleeve surgery, patients lose about 60-70% of excess weight in just a year. With exercise and proper eating, patients can lose even more weight in the coming years. Five years after surgery, on average, patients keep off over half of their extra weight. If you are diligent about diet, exercise, and doctor follow-ups, you can keep off all of it.

Can improve obesity-related diseases

When patients are sure to follow-up with their doctors following surgery, it's very common to see improvement in conditions like diabetes, hypertension, asthma, and more. Some even become cured. The benefits of maintaining a healthy weight cannot be overstated.

Less follow-up and risk of complications than other surgeries

For many, the most significant benefit of the gastric sleeve is less need for regular check-ups and less complications. Both gastric bypass and duodenal switch surgeries reduce the body's ability to absorb nutritions, so blood tests are *required* for the rest of your life to prevent malnutrition. Tests are still necessary following gastric sleeve, but the follow-up isn't as intense because gastric sleeve surgery does not inhibit nutrition absorption.

Also, because both bypass and duodenal switch surgeries are more complicated, your risk for issues like pain, bloating, digestion problems, and more increases. As for lap-band surgery, regular adjustments to the band are required, while the presence of a foreign object in the body (the silicone band itself) can cause issues.

Benefits of gastric sleeve surgery include a less complex procedure, less appetite, no dumping syndrome, significant weight loss, and less risks than other weight-loss surgeries.

WHEN TO GET GASTRIC SLEEVE SURGERY

There are requirements most patients need to meet in order to receive gastric sleeve surgery, including:

A BMI of 40+ *or*

A BMI between 30-39.9 and a obesity-related disease like high blood pressure, Type 2 diabetes, sleep apnea, or high cholesterol

POSSIBLE COMPLICATIONS

As with any surgery, gastric sleeve comes with possible complications. It's important to know what they are and their symptoms, so if you begin to suffer, you can seek medical attention right away:

Gallstones

Gallstones are one of the most reported complications after gastric sleeve surgery. Within two years, 23% of patients get gallbladder disease. Sometimes surgeons will even remove the gallbladder while performing the surgery. Symptoms of gallstones include pain in your upper back and abdomen, nausea, vomiting, indigestion, bloating, gas, and heartburn. If the pain can't be numbed by regular pain medication; you're vomiting; or you have chills, sweats, or a fever, you should go to the ER.

Staple line leaks

A week following surgery, surgeons are most worried about staple line leaks. They aren't common - about 2.4% are at risk - but they're very serious. Symptoms include an increased heart rate, trouble breathing, and a fever. If you experience any of these three, call your doctor. If it's been three days or less since your surgery, surgeons will go back in with a laparoscope and repair the leak. If it's been 8 days or longer, you most likely won't have to go through surgery. Other treatment such as stents and drainage are more common at this point.

Blood clots

A surgery is a type of injury - you are being cut into - and blood clots are always a risk with an injury. They also tend to occur when you don't move a lot after your injury, which will happen following surgery. Clots can be life-threatening, so getting attention quickly is vital. Symptoms include numbness, redness, swelling, pain, and paleness in your arm and legs.

Strictures

A stricture is when the opening to your stomach (the actual stomach, not your surgery scar opening) or to your intestines get inflamed or blocked. This prevents food from making its normal journey through the body. You might have a stricture if you feel nauseated, have trouble swallowing, you're vomiting, or you can't eat certain foods.

Wound site infection

After surgery, the areas where the surgeon made incision cuts can become infected. Infection is a risk that comes with every type of surgery. If your incision areas feel hot or look red, or you're experiencing a fever, faster heart rate, lightheadedness, or dizziness, you might have an infection.

SIDE EFFECTS

Complications are dangerous, but side effects are common post-surgery. Most of the time they aren't life-threatening; they're just annoying. However, you shouldn't ignore them since they may be symptoms of something more serious. Here are some of the discomforts patients tend to experience:

Nausea

You'll most likely feel nauseated during the first months following surgery. You might even need to vomit. Your body is doing a lot of healing and then adjusting to different foods.

Body aches

If these become too painful and you want to take a painkiller, ask your doctor which type is best. Common ones like Aleve and ibuprofen are usually *not* recommended.

Weakness and fatigue

Again, your body just went through a major surgery, so it needs rest. You're also consuming much less food, so your energy levels will be low.

Constipation

This happens because you aren't eating enough fiber. Drinking more fluids, taking fiber supplements, and walking can help.

Diarrhea or gas

You've most likely eaten something that's triggered stomach distress. Identify what you've eaten recently and then avoid it in the future.

Feeling cold

As you lose weight, you might feel colder than before. This is because fat insulates your body, and as you lose it, you lose that insulation.

Acne or dry skin

Some patients experience skin changes following weight-loss surgery. A healthy diet and the proper vitamins can help, as well as cleansers and lotions.

Hair loss

Hair loss is actually very common and occurs in 50% of patients following surgery. It happens because you are losing weight so quickly. The right diet, protein, and vitamins should help. You can also find special shampoos and supplements like flax seed oil.

Yeast infection

Antibiotics, which you take to prevent infection, can cause a yeast infection. Also known as thrush, this condition can result in a white coating on your tongue, redness, or inflammation. Talk to your doctor.

Moodiness

Feeling emotional after weight-loss surgery is very common. You might experience fear, anxiety, depression, uncertainty, or even regret. You might also feel frustrated about your recovery. The best solution is to stay connected to supportive friends and family and find peer support groups.

> **Complications of gastric-sleeve surgeries include gallstones, staple line leaks, blood clots, strictures, and wound site infections. Side effects, which are more common and usually less serious, include nausea, body aches, constipation, fatigue, and moodiness.**

II. WHAT TO DO *BEFORE* SURGERY

In the weeks before your surgery, your doctor will stay in close contact with you. You will undergo a health assessment, which includes questions about any medications you're taking, as well as your medical and surgical history. You get blood tests, X-rays, and an ECG, which measures the electrical activity of your heartbeat. The most significant "must-do," however, will be to change your diet.

How to eat

A change in diet can make your surgery much safer because it lowers your risk for complications. Obesity results in a large, fatty liver, which makes weight-loss surgeries like a gastric sleeve trickier for surgeons to perform. In the two weeks before surgery, you can actually shrink your liver with a diet change, making the surgery safer. Your pre-op diet will most likely consist of 800-1200 calories a day, which lets you lose weight. A diet change can also prepare you for your eating lifestyle post-surgery. Here's what most surgeons recommend:

Consume more protein

Think high-quality protein shakes that don't contain sugar. There are even shakes you can find designed specifically for bariatric patients, so they contain the nutrition you need to replace meals. Some patients may be able to eat lean, clean meats like chicken. Between 70-120 grams of protein is the common recommendation per day.

Eat less carbs

Avoid the refined carbs found in rice, cereal, pasta, bread, pizza, and potatoes. These high-calorie, heavy foods make losing weight and shrinking your liver harder. In place of carb-heavy meals, you'll be drinking most of your calories through protein shakes, broths, and soups.

Cut out sugar and foods high in fat

Sugar is the worst thing you can eat before weight-loss surgery. You will need to cut out all sweets, desserts, and fruit juice. It doesn't matter if you're drinking 100% fruit juice; natural fruit sugar is still sugar. Sugar-free snacks might be allowed very sparingly. High-fat foods are also bad for you before a gastric sleeve surgery, so cut out cheese, fatty meats, and all fried foods.

Drink more liquid

Adequate hydration is crucial to achieving and maintaining good health and weight loss. Also, when you feel hungry, you might actually be thirsty. You'll drink more than just water, because you need some nutrition. Bone broth, vegetable broth, and 100% vegetable juice will probably be recommended. These can also help with hunger. You aren't allowed to have caffeine, so if you drink tea or coffee, you have to go decaf with sugar-free sweeteners and soy, skim, or nut milk.

Two days before surgery

You'll need to be very strict with your diet two days before your surgery. Surgeons will probably tell you to stick to an all-clear liquid diet: broth, water, sugar-free Jello-O, water, and protein shakes, though you should only have one protein shake per day. Anything carbonated or caffeinated is off-limits. You should also consult with your surgeon about whether you should stop taking any medications you're currently on.

12 HOURS BEFORE

Twelve hours before your surgery, you shouldn't eat or drink anything. If you smoke, you should also refrain from any tobacco use.

SURGERY DAY

You won't eat or drink anything on surgery day. If you haven't had surgery before, you will enter the room and remove all your clothing and any jewelry. You'll put on the hospital gown and meet with the people performing your surgery. They'll hook you up to an IV and you'll get the medication that puts you under for the surgery.

> **Before surgery, your diet changes significantly. For 2-3 weeks before gastric sleeve surgery, you need to eat more protein, eat less carbs, cut out sugar and high-fat foods, and drink more liquid. 2 days before the surgery, you'll go on an all-clear liquid diet. 12 hours before, you stop eating and drinking completely.**

III. GUIDELINES AFTER GASTRIC SLEEVE SURGERY

There are two possible diet transitions that surgeons recommend: a conservative transition or an aggressive transition. For a conservative transition, you won't eat or drink *anything* the first day following your surgery. If the doctor determines an aggressive transition is best, you will begin with clear liquids on Day One, pureed foods on Day Two, and solid foods on Day Three. Conservative transitions are more common, however, where you don't add solid foods to your diet until Week Four or later. This is the method this cookbook follows.

For the conservative transition, your diet goes through four phases, each around a week long. This lets your body heal and recover from the gastric sleeve surgery, lowering your risk for complications. If you "cheat" during any of the four weeks, you might experience dehydration, constipation, bowel obstruction, diarrhea, or something much more serious. Let's break down the four-week post-op diet:

Week One - Clear liquids only

A diet of only clear liquids is challenging, but following gastric sleeve surgery, most patients don't really feel like eating. Your "food" will consist of:

- Water
- Clear vegetable, beef, or chicken broth
- Sugar-free Jello
- Sugar-free popsicles
- Decaf tea/coffee
- Unsweetened diluted juices without pulp

You won't be drinking anything sugary, caffeinated, or carbonated. It's also a good idea to avoid temperature extremes. For warm beverages, drink them in the morning since they relax the stomach muscles.

Week Two - Liquid diet w/ protein

Most patients will begin to feel hungry again during Week Two, but you'll still need to stick to a mostly-liquid diet. 64-ounces is the usual recommendation. Now, you can add a bit more protein, so you'll be drinking all your first week liquids *and:*

- Sugar-free pudding
- Soup with soft noodles
- Protein powder mixed with water or nut milks
- Non-fat yogurt
- Watered-down, no-sugar juice
- Watered-down hot oatmeal
- Sugar-free sorbet
- Sugar-free Carnation instant breakfasts
- Cream soups
- Cream of wheat

Keep in mind that some people don't handle dairy well after surgery, so be cautious. Some people even become lactose intolerant because of the sugar. Instead of regular dairy, you can use almond, coconut, or another milk.

Week Three - Pureed foods

You'll now begin to feel more normal, hunger-wise, so the temptation to cheat might kick in. However, you are not healed yet; it's very important to stick to your diet. You will need to get 60 grams of protein per day now and any new foods need to be introduced slowly and one at a time, so you can see how your body responds. If you keep vomiting and you're doing everything else right like eating slowly and eating very small amounts, you'll probably need to go back to Phase Two.

- During Week Three, you can now begin adding foods like:
- One protein shake a day
- Low-fat cottage cheese
- Softened, low or no-sugar cereals
- Steamed or boiled vegetables (avoid fibrous ones like celery, asparagus, raw leafy greens, and broccoli)
- Soup
- Scrambled eggs
- Soft steamed fish

- Canned fish
- Mashed bananas and avocados
- Low-sugar canned fruit
- Low or no-sugar smoothies

This is also the phase where you begin weighing your food. You want at least 12-ounces of food divided between three meals. At each meal, three ounces should be protein, with one ounce of a healthy fat. Two ounces can be a fruit or vegetable. Your protein shake counts as liquid, so it isn't weighed.

Week Four - Introducing solid foods

Finally, it's time for "real" food! You want to be cautious and always chew slowly. Your stomach and gastric sleeve are sensitive, so you still want to go for softer foods as your foundation. Three small meals a day with lots of hydration is best, though surgeons may let you have one small snack a day. Some might recommend eating five to six fist-sized meals a day instead; it depends on the surgeon and patient. You'll be introducing foods like:

- Fruit
- Softened vegetables (again avoiding fibrous ones)
- Fish
- Protein shakes
- Chicken
- Lean beef
- Sweet potatoes
- Mashed potatoes
- Baked potatoes
- Cereal
- Some caffeine

You still shouldn't have foods like candy, sweets, pastas, whole milk, dairy products, sodas, fried foods, and other high-carb items.

Diet guidelines past Week Four

Week Four is the last "official" recovery phase, but it isn't as if you can just go back to your old eating habits once that week ends. You'll continue introducing foods and monitoring how they make you feel. Here are some tips for Week Five and the future:

Continue eating three small meals a day, and maybe one healthy, nutrient-dense snack.

You don't want to start eating big meals or eating at random times just because Week Four is over. Your stomach has been transformed from what it was before, and the best eating style is still three-meals-a-day + one-snack. That's all you need. Be sure that you're getting 60 grams of protein daily.

Stay hydrated, but stop drinking one hour-30 minutes before eating a meal.

Surgeons will recommend drinking between 48-64 ounces a day. That's about eight cups. You want to drink slowly and gradually; chugging isn't good. Keep a drink with you and sip every 15-20 minutes. At this point, water isn't actually the best choice all the time; patient are often told to make water no more than half of their recommended liquid consumption. This is because water doesn't contain nutrients. Your other liquids can include bone broth, vegetable juice, diluted fruit juice, and herbal tea. Why stop drinking one hour before a meal? Filling your stomach with liquid can cause food to flush through your stomach too quickly, allowing you to overeat. You also shouldn't drink with your meal for the same reason.

Begin exercising daily.

You're in a good place to begin exercising now. Talk to your surgeon about what your activity level should be like. Generally, you will start with very basic movements as soon as you are able, like standing, sitting up, and focused, deep breathing. Walking comes next, followed by standing to take showers. Between weeks four and six, you can begin your usual exercises, including heavy lifting. Again, it depends on what your doctor recommends for your specific situation.

Don't drink soda or other sugary beverages.

This one is a give-in. Sugar has no nutritional value and can mess up your recovery really quickly. It's also highly-addictive and once you've given into a craving, you'll only want more. Soda also causes bloating, gas, and can inhibit the healing process. Non-carbonated drinks with sugar are just as bad. Just don't drink them.

> **After surgery, recovery is divided into four phases: clear liquids only, a liquid diet with protein shakes, pureed foods, and then the introduction of solid foods. Following the diet to the letter ensures you heal properly and don't experience complications.**

HOW TO GET MORE PROTEIN INTO YOUR DIET

Eating enough protein is crucial for your recovery, but it can be hard to get that big of an amount into your diet, especially when your diet is limited. There are three good ways to solve this problem: protein shakes, protein water, and protein bars.

Protein shakes

There are a lot of subpar protein shakes and powders out there. Many are too full of sugar and artificial ingredients. Some good brands include Premier Protein, Pure Protein, and Genepro.

Premier offers 30 grams of protein and 160 calories, with just one gram of sugar. There are also 24 vitamins and minerals. For variety, you can choose from flavors like chocolate, banana, strawberry & cream, or vanilla. It comes in both a powder form and premade shake form.

Pure Protein makes a Frosty Chocolate shake with 35 grams of protein, one gram of fat, and one gram of sugar per 170-calorie serving. Other flavors include banana cream, vanilla, strawberry, and cookies 'n cream. The powdered version has 25 grams of protein per 39-gram scoop and two grams of sugar.

Looking for something that's flavorless? Genepro is highly-recommended powder for bariatric patients. Per tablespoon, it has 30 grams of protein. It can be mixed into both hot or cold liquids.

Whenever you're choosing a shake, make sure it meets the following requirements:

- Less than 200 calories per serving
- At least 20 grams of protein per serving
- Less than 10 grams of sugar per serving
- No added sugar

Protein water

Protein water is a recent invention that infuses water with vitamins and protein. It doesn't have that thick, milky quality of protein shakes, so many people find it easier and more pleasant to drink. There are lots of brands hitting the market. Trimino, Protein 2o, Premier, and Isopure all make good waters.

Trimono contains 28 calories and seven grams of whey protein isolate. It's also packed with vitamins B3, B5, B6, and B12. It's sweetened with sucralose, so it has no carbs or sugar. Flavors include coconut pineapple, mixed berry, peach, and strawberry lemonade.

Protein 2o has a higher protein content than Trimono with 15 grams. That also means it's more calories, but it's still just 60 grams. It also has all 9 essential amino acids, so it's really good for workout recovery. Protein 2o contains just one carb and zero sugar grams; it's sweetened with sucralose. Flavors include mixed berry, grape, wild cherry, lemonade, and coconut.

Premier is also forging into the protein water business with a drink that has 20 grams of protein per 90-calorie serving. There's no sugar, two carbs, and no artificial flavors. For now, there are just two flavors: orange mango and raspberry. This is a slightly-creamy water, since it has a little bit of milk, but it's still much thinner than a protein shake.

Isopure has no grams of fat, sugar, and carbs. It contains 40 grams per 160-calorie serving, and is especially good for vegetarians, gluten-free dieters, and sugar-free dieters. There are lots of flavors, including orange, passion fruit, pineapple, coconut, and Alpine punch.

Protein bars

Protein bars are tricky because they're often no better than candy bars. There are a few that can be good meal replacements during Week Four or Five of your gastric-sleeve surgery recovery and as a snack in the future. Consider BariatricPal, Quest Nutrition, and Pure Protein.

BariatricPal protein bars are designed specifically for recovery from gastric sleeve or bypass surgery. They contain 15 grams of protein, six grams of fiber, and just five grams of sugar. One bar totals 160 calories. There are a handful of dessert-flavored options, though take note that some contain slightly more sugar and less protein than others.

Quest Nutrition offers a ton of flavors and are very low in sugar. One bar contains 20-21 grams of protein, one gram of sugar, and 14-17 grams of fiber. They do have 21 carbs, which is a bit high. Flavors include chocolate chip cookie dough, cinnamon, peanut butter, lemon, and raspberry. One bar equals 200 calories.

Pure Protein bars are gluten-free, and offer 20 grams of protein with just two grams of sugar, six grams of fat, and 17 carbs. Each bar is less than 200 calories. Flavors include chocolate peanut butter, chocolate deluxe, and chocolate peanut butter. The chocolate peanut butter has 20 grams of protein and two grams of sugar, making it the best choice of the three.

When looking at protein bars, don't only look at the protein count. Some bars have high protein, but also a lot of sugar. The bars above have the most protein and least sugar.

> **During week 4 when you're introducing solid foods and also in the long-term, getting enough protein can be challenging. Protein shakes, waters, and bars can be a good option if they're less than 200 calories per bar, have at least 20 grams of protein, and contain less than 10 grams of sugar.**

IV. GENERAL RECOVERY TIPS

Everyone's recovery journey is different following gastric sleeve surgery. You should always listen to the advice of your surgeon over anything you read in this book or online. To give you an idea of what your recovery is like, however, let's go through some general guidelines:

Expect constipation for the first week

In the section on side effects, we mentioned that constipation is common. It is most prevalent the week after your surgery. Pain medications are a contributing factor. Though it's considered normal, still talk to your doctor about it if it bothers you.

Take pain medication when you need it

There's nothing wrong with taking pain meds when you need them. Your doctor will prescribe you something. You should *never* take anything labeled as NSAIDs. This includes aspirin, Aleve, and ibuprofen. NSAIDs hinder the stomach's ability to produce mucous, which shields your stomach lining from gastric fluids. Surgeons might recommend an opioid like Vicodin or a acetaminophen-based medication, like Tylenol.

Walk as much as you can

For a while, the only exercise you'll be able to get is walking. Heavy lifting is dangerous, since it puts pressure on your stitches, and you'll likely be too tired to do anything strenuous. Walking encourages healing and establishes a good activity habit you can rely on in the future.

Don't take baths for three weeks

Hot baths can increase your risk for infection, because the heat can soften scabs and create an ideal environment for bacteria. You need to wait until the incisions are healed. This can take three weeks. Showers are usually okay, but consult with your surgeon first.

Depending on your job, you can expect to return in two to four weeks

If your job doesn't involve heavy lifting or strenuous physical activity, you can probably go back in two to four weeks. Your surgeon can help you decide if you are feeling well enough. Remember to keep walking around and avoid sitting too long. You'll also be avoiding those tempting office treats, so having a healthy snack option will be important.

Sip your liquids

Whatever liquid you're drinking, you want to *sip* it. No chugging. Drinking too quickly causes pain, bloating, and other unpleasant side effects. When you first get home, drinking may be difficult. Sipping keeps you hydrated, but comfortable. It's a good idea to aim for eight-ounces of liquid within 5-15 minutes for eight hours a day.

Eat small portions

Portion control is the second most important aspect of weight-loss after food choices. You can eat very healthy food, but if you're eating too much of it, you'll gain weight. To help with portion control, people often use small plates, cut up their food before they eat it, and/or use a kitchen scale to measure specific ounces. When you're starting to eat solid foods, you'll need to pay special attention to portions because you aren't sure what foods might bother you. Once you're fully healed, portion control ensures you keep losing weight.

Wear comfortable, loose clothing

Wearing tight clothing can make digestion uncomfortable. Pressure on your stomach actually inhibits the digestion process and can cause heartburn. When you're healing from gastric sleeve surgery, you want digestion to go as smoothly as possible. Wear clothing that's loose and comfortable. When you're recovering, you won't be going out, so loose sweatpants and pajama pants are completely acceptable.

Be patient

Recovering from surgery is frustrating. You might feel ready to eat solid food, and then suffer a setback. Maybe you really want to walk farther, but you are struggling with too much fatigue. You feel depressed or anxious. Your body affects your mental state and vice versa. The best thing you can do is to be patient with yourself. Not everyone heals and progresses in the same way, so don't compare yourself to others who've had gastric sleeve surgery. Monitor your mental health as closely as your physical health, and talk to your doctor if you're struggling. You might benefit from a counseling session or two.

> **When you're recovering from your surgery, it's a good idea to anticipate constipation, take pain meds when you need to, walk as much as you can, take showers instead of baths, slowly sip your liquids, and be patient with yourself. Depending on your job, you can expect to go back in 2-4 weeks after the gastric sleeve surgery.**

VITAMINS AND SUPPLEMENTS

Since you aren't eating a lot of food following gastric sleeve surgery, you will need to get nutrition from vitamins and supplements. With gastric sleeves, you don't need as many as you would with gastric bypass, but they're still necessary. Here's what a surgeon will typically recommend:

Multivitamin

A high-quality multivitamin is first on your list. Depending on the dose of each pill, you might take one in the morning and one at night. Brands for bariatric patients include Bariatric Fusion and Barimelts, though you can take other daily multivitamins.

Calcium citrate

You start taking this vitamin about 1 month following surgery. It's a three-a-day vitamin, and you should take it in 500 mg with at least 60 minutes between each dose. You should also take it two hours before or after your multivitamin and/or iron supplement. Iron and calcium cannot be mixed together. Calcium citrate can be taken with or without food.

Iron

If your doctor finds you need iron and you aren't getting enough from your multivitamin, you might be prescribed an additional iron supplement. It cannot be taken with calcium citrate, thus the two-hour window. Iron should be taken on an empty stomach; it's absorbed best this way.

Vitamin B12

Your doctor might recommend B12 injections, nasal sprays, or sublinguals (which means under the tongue). It can't be taken in pill form after surgery. The usual dose is between 5000-7500 mcg once a week.

Folate

If you have low folate levels, you are at risk for anemia. While multivitamins do contain folate, your doctor might recommend more if your levels are low. Ask to get tested every few months, since most surgeons don't automatically check.

Protein supplement

Getting 60 grams of protein daily can be tricky for those on a restricted diet. Surgeons will most likely recommend a protein supplement designed for bariatric patients. These include Genepro, Unjury, and Bariatric Fusion.

Getting enough nutrition is crucial to good health, so you'll likely need to take a multivitamin as well as calcium citrate, iron, vitamin B12, folate, and protein supplements.

V. STAYING ON TRACK FOLLOWING SURGERY

What are the secrets to success following a gastric sleeve surgery? There really aren't "secrets," per say, just good advice. Once your weeks of recovery are over, you don't stop the good habits you've developed. You'll still take your vitamins and supplements, eat healthy, and avoid unhealthy foods. *Note*: You may not need to continue taking supplements if you're getting enough from your diet, since gastric sleeves don't inhibit nutrition absorption. Stay in touch with your doctor about this.

There are steps you can take to make the long-term journey easier, like finding support groups, talking to a nutritionist, meal-planning, and more. Here are the best tips collected from blogs and experts:

Attend a support group

Support is very important whenever you're trying to meet a goal. Weight loss and good health is no exception. Having people who know what you're going through, are encouraging, and can walk with you on the journey are invaluable. Your hospital will have support group resources, so you can find people who are also recovering from bariatric patients. Having this accountability is very important in the long-term when you're able to eat more and need to make more decisions.

Limit or quit snacking

When your body has healed and you're adding solid foods back in, it can be tempting to start snacking again. Be very consistent about limiting yourself to just one healthy snack a day to get in enough protein, or stop altogether. Eating between meals is a really fast way to eat too many calories, and snack foods are frequently full of sugar, fat, and carbs.

Don't drink alcohol

Alcohol is packed with sugar and calories - just one gram equals 7.1 calories. Mixed drinks are the worst, because they have multiple types of alcohol. Booze is also likely to be stored as fat. Those are just the chemical components of alcohol; it can also make you emotional and more likely to indulge in unhealthy foods, because you won't have as much self-control. A glass of red wine every now and then with a nice dinner is just fine, but you should definitely cut out most drinking if you want to enjoy long-term success.

Slow down (eating and drinking)

A big reason for overeating is based on speed. When we eat quickly, we don't realize we're actually full until we feel *too* full. Slowing down lets us hear our bodies more clearly, and prevents effects like gas and bloating. It also lets us savor our food more.

Stick to high protein, low fat, low sugar

These are the three pillars of long-term eating after weight-loss surgery. You should always eat your protein source first, and it should be lean with excess fat removed. Vegetables and fruit should be your next priority, with carbs like potatoes, rice, and pasta coming in last. Always choose a food option with the lowest sugar.

Keep your blood sugar stable

We mentioned how you should eat three small meals a day and maybe one snack, but if your blood sugar needs require more than that, you should eat snacks. Choose carefully and consider what your meals look like - maybe you aren't including enough protein or another essential type of vitamin/mineral.

To enjoy long-term success following weight-loss surgery, there are many things you can do, including join a support group; avoid snacking and alcohol; stick to a high-protein, low-fat, low-sugar diet; meal plan; stay in touch with your doctor; and monitor your diet with a food journal of some kind.

Meal plan

Studies consistently show that people who plan their meals eat better and are less likely to overeat. Plan out your meals three to five days ahead, write down what ingredients you need, and then go shopping. It becomes easier to stick to what you need versus what looks tempting. You can also be intentional about the amount of calories each meal has, as well as the macronutrients like protein.

Keep in touch with your doctor

Your doctor is your most important resource following gastric sleeve surgery. You want to keep in close contact with them and tell them when you experience any pain or discomfort. They are the ones to test your vitamin and mineral levels, and prescribe any supplements or medications you might need. They can also refer you to other helpful resources. For the long-term, it is a good idea to get in touch with a nutritionist who specializes in bariatric patients. They have a more specific focus than a regular surgeon and can provide more help with food-related issues and questions.

Keep a diet journal

Monitoring your nutrition in the long-term is essential to keeping excess weight off. It's also vital to achieve good health, since you need to be aware of your mineral/vitamin levels. Studies have shown that those who keep food journals are twice as likely to lose more weight and keep it off.

For many people, an old-fashioned notebook and pen is good enough, but counting up your calories, protein grams, and more can be tedious if you're doing it longhand. Another option is to use an app. Baritastic is a great choice, since it's free and is designed for those who've had weight-loss surgery. Features include the standard food logs for whatever you eat and drink; vitamin/supplement reminders; recipes; photos; and connection to wearable fitness devices. The best feature, however, is that a doctor or nutritionist can actually sign in and access your data. This lets them check in on how you're doing and offer recommendations.

Stay positive

This is a rather vague cliche, but a positive mindset is crucial to long-term weight-loss success. What this means in practice is accepting your mistakes and flaws, but always seeking to learn from them and not give up. A positive mindset drives you forward and doesn't allow you to wallow in the past or negative thoughts. Maintaining this kind of upbeat attitude can be difficult, and there will be times when it seems impossible. Accept those down times, as well, and know that they will pass. If you experience more "lows" than "highs," it might be a good idea to consider counseling or seeking help from your support group and community.

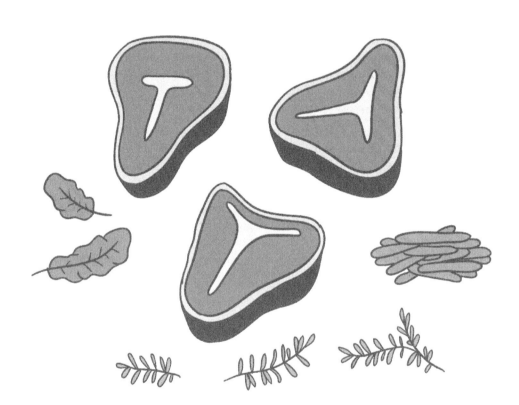

CHAPTER 1: WEEK 1-2 (FULL LIQUID, PHASE 1) (20)

Contents

Almond Tea

Servings: 4 / Preparation Time: 5 minutes/ Cooking Time: 5 minutes

Liquid drinks don't have to be bland right? This delicious almond tea will be the perfect way to start your day!

5 tablespoons almond powder

1 cup of water

1 teaspoon cinnamon

- Take a saucepan and place it over high heat, add water and stir in rest of the ingredients.
- Bring to a boil and remove heat.
- Serve and enjoy!

Per Serving: Calories: 40; Total Fat: 3g; Saturated Fat: 0g; Protein: 1.5g; Carbs: 1.4g; Fiber: 0.1g

Alcohol-Free Mint Mojito

Servings: 4 / Preparation Time: 5 minutes/ Cooking Time: 30 minutes

Just because you had the surgery, doesn't mean that you have to get rid of all the good stuff from your life right? This Alcohol-Free Mojito is the perfect drink for you!

12/2 cup fresh mint leaves	½ cup natural sweetener
1-ounce lime juice	2 cups of water

- Add water and sweetener in a pot and let it boil for 5 minutes until the syrup has thickened.
- Transfer mint leaves in a glass jar and pours in the syrup.
- Cover jar and let it steep for 20 minutes.
- Create a mixture of a tablespoon of the syrup and half a cup of cold water in a glass, add lime juice and mix, serve and enjoy!

Per Serving: Calories: 32; Total Fat: 0g; Saturated Fat: 0g; Protein: 0g; Carbs: 3g; Fiber: 1g

Sugar-Free Strawberry Limeade

Servings: 4 / Preparation Time: 5 minutes/ Cooking Time: 30 minutes

Mix up strawberry and lime, and you will have the perfect strawberry flavored limeade to go for!

½ teaspoon strawberry extract   Juice of ½ a lime

1 and ½ cups cold water

- Mix in strawberry extract, lime juice and water in a bowl.
- Take a cup and add ice cubes, pour the strawberry mixture and enjoy!

Per Serving: Calories: 12; Total Fat: 0g; Saturated Fat: 0g; Protein: 1g; Carbs: 2.1g; Fiber: 0.5g

Hearty Mint Tea

Servings: 4 / Preparation Time: 5 minutes/ Cooking Time: 30 minutes

This one for those who are looking for a more soothing effect in their tea as opposed to a warm and hearty feeling. Perfect to heal cough as well.

1 gallon boiling water

2 tablespoons mint

1 lemon, sliced

6 Rooibos tea bags

- Place water over high heat and let it start boiling.
- Remove heat and add tea bags.
- Pour the mixture into a pitcher (alongside teabags, mint and sliced lemon) and let it steep for 30 minutes.
- Serve and enjoy!

Per Serving: Calories: 4; Total Fat: 0g; Saturated Fat: 0g; Protein: 0.1g; Carbs: 1.4g; Fiber: 0.1g

Kiwi Sorbet

Servings: 4 / Preparation Time: 5 minutes/ Cooking Time: nil

A delicious sorbet made of orange and Kiwi, refreshing and yummy!

4 and ½ cups crushed ice cubes

½ pound kiwi fruit, chopped

1 tablespoon orange zest, grated

- Add listed ingredients to your blender.
- Blend for 30 seconds.
- Serve and enjoy!

Per Serving: Calories: 105; Total Fat: 0.3g; Saturated Fat: 0g; Protein: 0.6g; Carbs:26g; Fiber: 0.1g

Orange Vanilla Tea

Servings: 4 / Preparation Time: 10 minutes/ Cooking Time: 5 minutes

The vanilla extract used in this drink will give a very fine fragrance to this orange delight.

¼ cup of water

2 oranges, sliced

¼ teaspoon vanilla extract

- Take a saucepan and place it over high heat, add all of the mixtures and bring to a boil.
- Remove heat and let it sit for 5 minutes.
- Strain the mixture and serve, enjoy!

Per Serving: Calories: 60; Total Fat: 1g; Saturated Fat: 0g; Protein: 2g; Carbs: 14g; Fiber: 0.1g

Orange And Apricot Juice

Servings: 2 / Preparation Time: 10 minutes/ Cooking Time: nil

Taking things up a notch, mixing in the apricot into the orange drink alongside an assorted collection of other items, does not only increase its flavor but also the health factor as well!

2 large oranges, peeled

2 large apricots, pitted

1 cup pomegranate seeds

1 cup of green grapes

1 large lemon, peeled

1 small ginger slice, peeled

- Peel oranges and divide them into wedges.
- Keep it on the side.
- Wash apricots and cut them in half, remove pits and cut them into small pieces.
- Cut the top of pomegranate fruit using a sharp knife and slice down each of the white membranes inside the fruit.
- Pop seeds into a measuring cup and keep it on the side.
- Peel lemon and cut it lengthwise in half and keep it on the side.
- Peel ginger slices and keep it on the side.
- Add orange, apricots, pomegranate, lemon ginger to a juicer and process until well juiced.
- Chill for 20 minutes and enjoy!

Per Serving: Calories: 196; Total Fat: 0.8g; Saturated Fat: 0g; Protein: 4g; Carbs: 48g; Fiber: 6.9g

Chicken Bone Broth

Servings: 4 / Preparation Time: 10 minutes/ Cooking Time: 2 hours

A simple warm and hearty chicken broth, no fuss and health inducing.

1 ounce of chicken bones

2 tablespoons apple cider vinegar

1 onion, sliced

6 garlic cloves

1 tablespoon cooking oil

½ teaspoon salt

½ teaspoon white pepper

1-inch ginger, sliced

Water

- Take a large skillet and add bones, water, onion, garlic, oil, ginger, vinegar, salt , pepper and gently stir.
- Cover with lid and cook on low heat for 2 hours.
- Strain the broth and discard any residue.
- Serve hot and enjoy!

Per Serving: Calories: 147; Total Fat: 5g; Saturated Fat: 0g; Protein: 10g; Carbs: 9g; Fiber: 0.5g

Apple And Citrus Juice

Servings: 2 / Preparation Time: 10 minutes/ Cooking Time: nil

A very cool apple juice packed with pinches of citrusy flavors coming from lemon, with a gentle heat from the ginger.

1 cup avocado, pitted and chopped

1 large cucumber, sliced

1 large lemon, peeled

1 cup fresh spinach, torn

1 large lime, peeled

1 small ginger knob, peeled

3 ounces of water

- Peel your avocado and cut it in half. Remove pit and chop the avocado into chunks.

- Wash cucumber and cut it into thick slices.

- Keep it on the side.

- Peel lemon and lime, cut it length in half.

- Wash your spinach thoroughly and tear it into small parts.

- Take your juicer and add avocado, cucumber, lemon, lime, spinach, ginger, and process until finely juiced.

- Let it chill for 20 minutes, serve and enjoy!

Per Serving: Calories: 197; Total Fat: 14g; Saturated Fat: 3g; Protein: 3g; Carbs: 19g; Fiber: 8g

Blueberry Mint Juice

Servings: 2 / Preparation Time: 10 minutes/ Cooking Time: nil

Fantastic Blueberry Juice accented by a minty flavor, amazing!

1 cup blueberries

1 cup fresh mint, torn

1 large red apple, cored

1 large cucumber, sliced

2 ounces of coconut water

- Prepare all the fruits and veggies accordingly.
- Wash them thoroughly and drain them, transfer everything to your juicer and process well until thoroughly juiced.
- Refrigerate for 15 minutes and add some ice, enjoy!

Per Serving: Calories: 145; Total Fat: 1g; Saturated Fat: 0g; Protein: 3.4g; Carbs: 35g; Fiber: 8.5g

Hearty Ginger Aid Juice

Servings: 2 / Preparation Time: 5 minutes/ Cooking Time: nil

A very hearty Oatmeal and Banana Smoothie, a perfect breather for phase 2!

1 bunch kale

½ bunch parsley

Green apple, seeded and cut

2-inch piece ginger

1 garlic clove, peeled

1 lemon, peeled

1 whole cucumber, ends removed

- Add listed ingredients to the blender and blend until the ingredients are blended and smooth.

- Pass through a fine mesh and extract the juice. Serve and enjoy!

- Alternatively, you may use a juicer if you have.

Per Serving: Calories: 79; Total Fat: 0g; Saturated Fat: 0g; Protein: 2g; Carbs: 18g; Fiber: 2g

Carrot And Coconut Broth

Servings: 4 / Preparation Time: 15 minutes/ Cooking Time: 20 minutes

If you are bored with the everyday simple broth, then this healthy veggie broth is the one to go for!

6 large carrots, thinly sliced

2 cups of coconut milk

1 medium-sized sweet potato, chopped

1 small onion, chopped

2 cups chicken broth

1 teaspoon curry powder

2 garlic cloves, crushed

1 tablespoon vegetable oil

1 teaspoon salt

¼ teaspoon black pepper, ground

- Take a deep pot and place it over medium-high heat, add olive oil and let it heat up.
- Add onions and stir fry until translucent. Add garlic and mix well, cook for 1 minute.
- Add carrots, potatoes, chicken broth and bring to a boil.
- Sprinkle curry powder, salt, and pepper. Cook for 15 minutes and add coconut milk.
- Cook until heated thoroughly.
- Separate broth and vegetables by passing the broth through a fine metal mesh or strainer.
- Serve and enjoy!

Per Serving: Calories: 271; Total Fat: 21g; Saturated Fat: 0g; Protein: 4.7g; Carbs: 17g; Fiber: 4g

Watercress Celery Juice

Servings: 1 / Preparation Time: 10 minutes/ Cooking Time: nil

A fine mixture of Celery and Watercress to fresh up your mood!

2 cups fresh watercress, chopped

2 large celery stalks, chopped

1 cup cucumber, sliced

1 whole lime, peeled

¼ teaspoon turmeric, ground

1 ounce of water

- Add watercress in a large colander, rinse thoroughly under cold water.
- Tear with hands and keep it on the side.
- Wash celery stalks and cut into bite-sized pieces.
- Wash cucumber and cut into thin slices.
- Fill measuring cup and keep reserve remaining cucumbers.
- Peel lime and cut lengthwise in half.
- Keep it on the side.
- Add watercress, celery, cucumber, lime in juicer and process well.
- Transfer to serving glass and stir in turmeric, water.
- Refrigerate for 10 minutes, enjoy!

Per Serving: Calories: 61; Total Fat: 0.8g; Saturated Fat: 0g; Protein: 3.9g; Carbs: 12g; Fiber: 4g

Pork Bone Broth

Servings: 4 / Preparation Time: 10 minutes/ Cooking Time: 2 hours

This one is for those of you who prefer to walk the pork side and enjoy a porky broth.

1 ounce pork bones

2 tablespoons apple cider vinegar

1 onion, sliced

6 garlic cloves

1 tablespoon cooking oil

½ teaspoon salt

½ teaspoon white pepper

1-inch ginger, sliced

Water

- Take a large skillet and add bones, water, onion, garlic, oil, ginger, vinegar, salt, pepper and gently stir.
- Cover with lid and cook on low heat for 2 hours.
- Strain the broth and discard any residue.
- Serve hot and enjoy!

Per Serving: Calories: 147; Total Fat: 5g; Saturated Fat: 0g; Protein: 10g; Carbs: 9g; Fiber: 0.5g

Hearty Lemon Balm Tea

Servings: 4 / Preparation Time: 5 minutes/ Cooking Time: 5 minutes

Hearty lemon balm tea to soothe your soul and energize your body.

1 cup lemon balm   1 tablespoon lemon zest

5 cups of water

- Add water to a pot and bring it to a boil.

- Add lemon balm, lemon zest, and stir.

- Remove the heat and let it cool.

- Strain and serve, enjoy!

Per Serving: Calories: 13; Total Fat: 0g; Saturated Fat: 0g; Protein: 0g; Carbs: 13g; Fiber: 0.1g

Basil And Blueberry Juice

Servings: 1 / Preparation Time: 10 minutes/ Cooking Time: nil

Absolutely smashing blueberry and basil juice to help you keep your flavor buds in check during the early phase days.

1 cup blueberries

1 cup fresh basil, torn

1 cup strawberries, sliced

1 whole lemon, peeled

1 small Granny Smith apple, cored

- Transfer blueberries to a colander and rinse under cold water, slightly drain and keep it on the side.
- Wash basil thoroughly and tear.
- Wash strawberries and remove stems, cut into slices and fill a measuring cup.
- Peel lemon and cut lengthwise in half. Keep it on the side.
- Wash apples and cut in half, remove core and cut into bite-sized pieces.
- Add blueberries, basil, strawberries, lemon, apple in a juicer and process until juiced well.
- Transfer to a glass and add ice cubes, enjoy!

Per Serving: Calories: 193; Total Fat: 1.3g; Saturated Fat: 0g; Protein: 3.5g; Carbs: 49g; Fiber: 11g

Red Apple And Carrot Tea

Servings: 4 / Preparation Time: 10 minutes/ Cooking Time: 5 minutes

We all love carrot juice, right? But have you ever tried apple and carrot tea? Trust me, it's amazing!

1 cup red apples, peeled and chunked

2 carrots, sliced

½ cup lychee, seeded

2 cups of water

- Blend apples with carrots, lychee, and water in a blender.
- Take a saucepan and place it over medium-high heat, add the listed ingredients to the pan alongside the blended mixture and bring the whole mixture to a boil.
- Remove heat and let it rest for 5 minutes.
- Strain and enjoy!

Per Serving: Calories: 184; Total Fat: 0g; Saturated Fat: 0g; Protein: 1g; Carbs: 9g; Fiber: 0.1g

Icy Banana Pops

Servings: 4 / Preparation Time: 4 hours 30 minutes/ Cooking Time: nil

Simple and easy banana flavored Ice Pops, perfect for you and even your kids!

1 cup boiling water

1 pack Jell-O, fruit flavored

1 banana

1 cup plain yogurt

- Add listed ingredients to a blender and blend until smooth.
- Pour mixture into Popsicle mold and let it freeze until hard.
- Serve and enjoy!

Per Serving: Calories: 93; Total Fat: 0.4g; Saturated Fat: 0g; Protein: 2.2g; Carbs: 22g; Fiber: 0.5g

Watermelon Sorbet

Servings: 4 / Preparation Time: 5 minutes/ Cooking Time: nil

The classic summertime breather!

4 and ½ cups crushed ice cubes   1 tablespoon orange zest, grated

½ pound melon, cubed

- Add listed ingredients to a blender and blend for 30 seconds.
- Serve and enjoy!

Per Serving: Calories: 231; Total Fat: 0.2g; Saturated Fat: 0g; Protein: 0.6g; Carbs: 59g; Fiber: 0.1g

Mustard And Tomato Green Juice

Servings: 1 / Preparation Time: 10 minutes/ Cooking Time: nil

This might sound like an odd combination at first, but in the long run, you will slowly learn to appreciate its health factor and warm and tangy flavor.

1 medium-sized Roma tomatoes, chopped

1 cup mustard greens, torn

1 cup fresh spinach, torn

1 large carrot, sliced

1 teaspoon fresh rosemary, finely chopped

- Wash tomato and transfer to a bowl.
- Cut into bite-sized pieces and make sure to reserve tomato juice while cutting.
- Wash mustard greens and spinach by running under cold water.
- Drain and tear with hands.
- Wash carrots and peel them, cut into thin slices.
- Add tomato, mustard greens, spinach, carrot, rosemary in a juicer and process until well juiced.
- Transfer to serving glass and stir in reserved tomato juice.
- Refrigerate for 15 minutes, enjoy!

Per Serving: Calories: 66; Total Fat: 0.5g; Saturated Fat: 0g; Protein: 3g; Carbs: 14g; Fiber: 5g

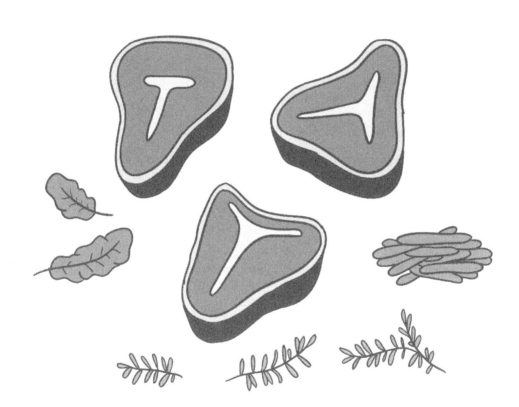

CHAPTER 2: WEEK 3 (PUREED FOODS AND SMOOTHIE, PHASE 2) (20)

Contents

Cucumber And Avocado Dill Smoothie

Servings: 2 / Preparation Time: 5 minutes/ Cooking Time: nil

A find dill and avocado smoothie to kick start your phase 2!

1 cucumber, peeled and sliced

2 tablespoons dill, chopped

2 tablespoons lemon juice

1 avocado, pitted

1 cup of coconut milk

1 teaspoon coconut, shredded

2 kiwis, peeled and sliced

- Take a blender and add all of the listed ingredients and blend well.
- Drain the extract and strain, discard any residue.
- Serve and enjoy!

Per Serving: Calories: 165; Total Fat: 5g; Saturated Fat: 1g; Protein: 2g; Carbs: 24g; Fiber: 0.1g

Pureed Salsa And Beans

Servings: 3 / Preparation Time: 5 minutes/ Cooking Time: 10 minutes

Just because you had the surgery doesn't mean that you have to get rid of beans from your diet! They are excellent sources of protein and this puree alone is a protein-packed punch!

1 scoop unflavored whey protein powder

2 tablespoons chicken broth

2 tablespoons salsa, your choice

15 ounces pinto beans

- Add listed ingredients in a small pot and let it heat up over medium-high heat.
- Gently stir until everything is warmed thoroughly.
- Pour mixture into a blender and puree for a few minutes until smooth.
- Transfer to serving the dish and enjoy!

Per Serving: Calories: 95; Total Fat: 0.4g; Saturated Fat: 0g; Protein: 11g; Carbs: 12g; Fiber: 0.5g

Pureed Kale Curry

Servings: 6 / Preparation Time: 10 minutes/ Cooking Time: 20 minutes

Fancy Pureed Kale dish, excellent if you are hungry during your phase 2 days.

2 cups kale leaves, chopped

2 cups chicken broth

1 teaspoon garlic paste

2-inch ginger sliced, shredded

¼ teaspoon turmeric powder

¼ teaspoon salt

1 green chili

1 tablespoon coconut oil

½ cup of water

- Take a blender and add kale, water, green chili and blend till pureed.
- Heat oil in a pan and place it over medium heat, add ginger and garlic and Sauté for 1 minute.
- Add kale and fry for 5 minutes.
- Pour chicken broth and add salt, cook on low for 15-20 minutes.

Per Serving: Calories: 269; Total Fat: 6g; Saturated Fat: 2g; Protein: 7g; Carbs: 48g; Fiber: 12g

Double Fudge Chocolate Shake

Servings: 2 / Preparation Time: 5 minutes/ Cooking Time: nil

The ultimate shake for chocolate lovers! Just give it a try and I can guarantee that you will fall for it.

1 cup low-fat milk

½ cup low-fat plain Greek yogurt

¼ cup chocolate protein powder

2 tablespoons unsweetened cocoa powder

½ small bananas

½ teaspoon vanilla extract

- Take your blender and add milk, yogurt, protein powder, cocoa powder, banana, vanilla and blend on high for 2-3 minutes.
- One the shake is smooth and the powders are dissolved, pour half the shake into a glass and enjoy!

Per Serving: Calories: 157; Total Fat: 1g; Saturated Fat: 0g; Protein: 20g; Carbs: 18g; Fiber: 3g

Coco Banana Milkshake

Servings: 2 / Preparation Time: 5 minutes/ Cooking Time: nil

A Mesmerizing coconut and banana shake, absolutely delightful! Plus the addition of cardamom adds a very warm flavor to the smoothie.

1 cup of coconut milk

2 ripe bananas

2 tablespoons cinnamon

¼ teaspoon cardamom powder

2 scoops protein powder

7 ice cubes

- Take a blender and add coconut milk, cardamom powder, cinnamon, bananas and blend the mixture well.
- Pour the mixture into glass and add ice chunks.
- Serve and enjoy!

Per Serving: Calories: 191; Total Fat: 7g; Saturated Fat: 1g; Protein: 25g; Carbs: 35g; Fiber: 0.1g

Fine Apple And Cucumber Juice

Servings: 4 / Preparation Time: 5 minutes/ Cooking Time: nil

A very refreshing and invigorating cucumber juice that brings a fine sweetness from the apple.

Head of 1 romaine lettuce

3 small mandarin oranges

Lime as needed

1 large lemon

1 large cucumber

3 medium apples

- Wash all the vegetables and fruits thoroughly.
- Add the fruits to your juicer (including skin) and juice them thoroughly.
- Serve and enjoy!

Per Serving: Calories: 146; Total Fat: 0.8g; Saturated Fat: 0g; Protein: 2g; Carbs: 11g; Fiber: 0g

Simple Healthy Soup

Servings: 4 / Preparation Time: 5 minutes/ Cooking Time: 10 minutes

Nothing too fancy here, just a simple and healthy soup packed with an assorted selection of veggies.

14 ounces cauliflower head, cut into florets

5 ounces watercress

7 ounces spinach, thawed

1 cup of coconut milk

¼ cup ghee

Salt and pepper to taste

1 onion, chopped

2 garlic cloves, crushed

- Grease Dutch oven with ghee and place it over medium-high heat.
- Add onion and garlic, cauliflower florets and cook for 5 minutes.
- Add spinach and watercress, cook for 2 minutes, add coconut milk.
- Pour vegetable stock and bring to a boil.
- Season with salt and pepper let it cool.
- Puree the soup and strain through a sieve, serve and enjoy!

Per Serving: Calories: 392; Total Fat: 37g; Saturated Fat: 0g; Protein: 4g; Carbs: 10g; Fiber: 0.1g

Guava Smoothie

Servings: 4 / Preparation Time: 5 minutes/ Cooking Time: nil

A fine Guava Smoothie to die for!

1 cup guava, seeds removed and chopped

1 cup baby spinach, finely chopped

1 banana, peeled and sliced

1 teaspoon fresh ginger, grated

½ medium sized mango, peeled and chopped

2 cups of water

- Peel guava and cut it in half, scoop out seeds and thoroughly wash it.
- Cut into small portions and keep it on the side.
- Rinse baby spinach under cold water and tear into small portions.
- Peel the banana and chop it up into small chunks. Keep it on the side.
- Peel Mango and cut it into small pieces, keep it on the side.
- Add guava, baby spinach, banana, ginger, mango to the juicer and process until well mixed and creamy.
- Transfer to a glass and let it chill for 20 minutes, serve and enjoy!

Per Serving: Calories: 166; Total Fat: 1.4g; Saturated Fat: 0.3g; Protein: 3.9g; Carbs: 39g; Fiber: 1g

Italian Chicken Puree

Servings: 1 / Preparation Time: 10 minutes/ Cooking Time: 1 minute

If you are in the mood to enjoy the essence of Italy, this simple Italian chicken puree is the one you should go for!

1 teaspoon Italian seasoning

Salt and pepper to taste

1 and ½ tablespoons tomato sauce

¼ cup of canned chicken

- Add listed ingredients to blender and pulse until the mixture is well incorporated.
- Use back of the fork to blend everything.
- Transfer to a bowl and microwave for 30 seconds.
- Enjoy!

Per Serving: Calories: 73; Total Fat: 4g; Saturated Fat: 3g; Protein: 13g; Carbs: 3g; Fiber: 0.5g

Mashed Cauliflower

Servings: 4 / Preparation Time: 5 minutes/ Cooking Time: 5 minutes

The classical cauliflower mash, perfect for every occasion!

1 large cauliflower head

¼ cup of water

1/3 cup low-fat buttermilk

1 tablespoon garlic, minced

1 tablespoon extra-virgin olive oil

- Break cauliflower into small florets.
- Place in a large microwave-safe bowl with water.
- Cover and microwave for 5 minutes, until cauliflowers are tender.
- Puree buttermilk, cauliflower, garlic, olive oil on medium speed on a food processor until the mixture is smooth.
- Enjoy!

Per Serving: Calories: 62; Total Fat: 2g; Saturated Fat: 0g; Protein: 3g; Carbs: 8g; Fiber: 2g

Pumpkin Spice Latte Protein Shake

Servings: 2 / Preparation Time: 5 minutes/ Cooking Time: nil

A protein-packed latte shake! Unique right? Tastes awesome too.

1 cup low-fat milk

½ cup pumpkin puree

½ cup vanilla protein powder

¾ cup brewed decaf coffee

1 teaspoon ground cinnamon

¼ teaspoon ground ginger

¼ teaspoon ground nutmeg

1/8 teaspoon ground cloves

- Take a blender and add milk, pumpkin puree, protein powder, coffee, cinnamon, ginger, nutmeg, and cloves.
- Blend on HIGH for 2-3 minutes until smooth.
- Pour half shake into a glass and enjoy!

Per Serving: Calories: 125; Total Fat: 0g; Saturated Fat: 0g; Protein: 15g; Carbs: 12g; Fiber: 2g

Chia Blueberry Banana Oatmeal Smoothie

Servings: 2 / Preparation Time: 5 minutes/ Cooking Time: nil

A very hearty Oatmeal and Banana Smoothie, a perfect breather for phase 2!

1 cup of soy milk

1 banana, sliced

¼ cup frozen blueberries

¼ cup oats

1 teaspoon vanilla extract

1 teaspoon cinnamon

1 tablespoon chia seeds

- Add listed ingredients to the blender and blend until the ingredients are blended and smooth.
- Serve and enjoy!

Per Serving: Calories: 178; Total Fat: 4g; Saturated Fat: 1g; Protein: 3g; Carbs: 36g; Fiber: 0.1g

Easy Spinach Dip

Servings: 2 / Preparation Time: 10 minutes + 2 hours chill time/ Cooking Time: nil

The easy and creative cheesy spinach dip, you'll fall in love with it!

1 cup plain non-fat Greek yogurt

4 ounces Neufchatel cheese

½ cup olive oil based mayonnaise

2 teaspoons garlic, minced

1 and ½ teaspoons onion powder

1 teaspoon smoked paprika

¾ teaspoon freshly ground black pepper

¼ teaspoon red pepper flakes

2 teaspoons Worcestershire sauce

1 (8 ounces) can water chestnuts, drained and finely chopped

½ cup scallions, chopped

1 (10 ounces) pack frozen spinach, chopped, thawed and squeezed

- Take a large bowl and yogurt, cheese, mayonnaise, garlic, onion powder, paprika, pepper, red pepper flakes, and sauce, mix on low speed using a hand mixer.
- Add water, chestnuts, scallions, spinach, and stir by hand.
- Cover and let it chill for 2 hours.
- Serve with veggies and enjoy!

Per Serving: Calories: 71; Total Fat: 4g; Saturated Fat: 0g; Protein: 3g; Carbs: 5g; Fiber: 1g

Smashed Potato Salad

Servings: 6 / Preparation Time: 10 minutes/ Cooking Time: nil

Potatoes are essentially one of the most universally acclaimed veggies ever to exist! Smashing them is the perfect way to enjoy them during phase 2.

3 pounds potatoes, quartered, boiled and mashed

4 eggs, hard-boiled, sliced

1 stalk celery, chopped

6 radishes, thinly sliced

2 tablespoons sweet pickle relish

3 green onions, sliced

¾ cup miracle whips dressing

1 tablespoon white vinegar

½ teaspoon paprika

- Add potatoes into a bowl while still warm, add remaining ingredients and combine well until mushy and fluffy.
- Serve and enjoy!

Per Serving: Calories: 204; Total Fat: 9g; Saturated Fat: 2g; Protein: 5g; Carbs: 25g; Fiber: 10g

Cherry And Mango Smoothie

Servings: 1 / Preparation Time: 10 minutes/ Cooking Time: nil

A hearty mango smoothie with added flavors from the cherry, yum.

¾ cup of water

1 cup of frozen mango, cubed

½ cup additional water

1 cup sweetened cherries, frozen

- Let the mangoes and cherries sit in separate bowls and let them thaw.
- Add cherries to blender with half a cup of water, blend until smooth.
- Pour the mixture into a glass.
- Rinse blender and add in mango alongside remaining water.
- Blend until smooth and pour mixture over cherries.
- Enjoy!

Per Serving: Calories: 185; Total Fat: 0g; Saturated Fat: 0g; Protein: 2g; Carbs: 46g; Fiber: 0.1g

Ginger Peach Smoothie

Servings: 4 / Preparation Time: 5 minutes/ Cooking Time: nil

Very warm and spicy flavors come from the ginger in this smoothie but are well balanced by the sweetness of the peach.

1 cup of coconut milk

1 large peach, chopped

1 tablespoon coconut oil

1 tablespoon chia seeds

1 teaspoon fresh ginger, peeled

- Wash your peach thoroughly and cut it into the half.
- Remove the pic and chop it into bite-sized portions, keep it on the side.
- Cut the small ginger knob, gently peel and chop it.
- Add peach, ginger, coconut milk, coconut oil in a blender and process until well blended.
- Serve and enjoy!

Per Serving: Calories: 201; Total Fat: 19g; Saturated Fat: 5g; Protein: 2.5g; Carbs: 8g; Fiber: 0g

Fresh Mango Smoothie

Servings: 4 / Preparation Time: 5 minutes/ Cooking Time: nil

A simple, no fuss mango smoothie with an added flavor from the coconut milk.

A handful of ice cubes

1 teaspoon vanilla extract, sugar-free

1 tablespoon walnuts, chopped

1 cup of coconut milk

1 medium mango, roughly chopped

- Peel the mango and cut it up into small chunks.
- Add mango, coconut milk, walnuts, vanilla extract to your blender. Blend well until smoothie.
- Stir in vanilla extract and add ice cubes, enjoy!

Per Serving: Calories: 271; Total Fat: 21g; Saturated Fat: 6g; Protein: 3g; Carbs: 21g; Fiber: 1g

Simple Oven-Baked Ricotta

Servings: 1 / Preparation Time: 10 minutes/ Cooking Time: 20 minutes

A fancy oven baked Ricotta recipe, awesome!

1 teaspoon Dijon mustard	¼ cup 2% cheddar cheese
1 teaspoon ground thyme	¼ cup reduced fat parmesan
1 whole egg	½ cup low-fat ricotta cheese

- Pre-heat your oven to 400 degrees F.
- Add listed ingredients in a bowl and mix well until the mixture is well combined.
- Use a cookie scoop and divide the mixture between 4 muffin tin cups.
- Slide into oven and bake for 20 minutes.
- Serve and enjoy!

Per Serving: Calories: 69; Total Fat: 4g; Saturated Fat: 1g; Protein: 8g; Carbs: 4g; Fiber: 0.1g

Authentic Orange Puree

Servings: 4 / Preparation Time: 5 minutes/ Cooking Time: 20 minutes

The perfect mixture of orange and carrots, this puree has the perfect balance of sweetness and citrus! You'll love it.

1 medium sweet potato, coarsely chopped   2 to 3 tablespoons of fresh water

3 medium carrots, cut into chunks

- Add potatoes and carrots to a medium sized pot and add water, bring the water over boil.
- Let it cook for 20 minutes until the veggies are tender.
- Drain the vegetables and transfer to a food processor, add 2 tablespoons of water.
- Puree on HIGH and serve, enjoy!

Per Serving: Calories: 364; Total Fat: 12g; Saturated Fat: 2g; Protein: 6g; Carbs: 50g; Fiber: 12g

Frozen Mocha Frappuccino

Servings: 4 / Preparation Time: 5 minutes/ Cooking Time: nil

The amazing chocolate Mocha Frappuccino! No longer do you have to go fast food joints to enjoy your daily dose of Sleeve Surgery friendly frap!

Low-sugar chocolate syrup as needed

Low-fat whipped cream as needed

1 cup ice

1 tablespoon cocoa powder

3-4 drops liquid sweetener

½ cup 0% fat Greek yogurt

¼ cup unsweetened almond milk

¼ cup brewed coffee

- Add ice, cocoa, sweetener, yogurt, milk, coffee to the blender and pulse well.
- Pour Frappuccino and top with whipped cream and chocolate syrup if needed.
- Enjoy!

Per Serving: Calories: 93; Total Fat: 2.7g; Saturated Fat: 0g; Protein: 11g; Carbs: 4g; Fiber: 0.8g

Hearty Black Bean And Lime Puree

Servings: 4 / Preparation Time: 5 minutes/ Cooking Time: 10 minutes

Very tasty and protein-packed bean and lime puree. The tenderness and meaty flavor of this recipe are to die for.

1 tablespoon unflavored protein powder

¼ cup vegetable broth

½ tablespoon jarred jalapeno juice

½ tablespoon lime juice

¼ cup rinsed black beans

- Once you have washed and rinsed your black beans, transfer to a small pot.
- Let them heat over medium heat.
- Mix in juice from jalapenos and lime juice, stir well and let it heat thoroughly.
- Once done, mix in chicken broth and pour the mixture into the blender.
- Mix gently until smooth.(Use an immersion blender if possible)
- Let the puree cool and mix in protein powder, enjoy!

Per Serving: Calories: 180; Total Fat: 2g; Saturated Fat: 0g; Protein: 30g; Carbs: 11g; Fiber: 1g

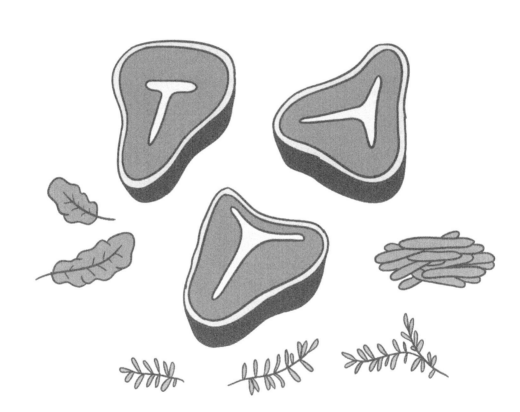

CHAPTER 3: WEEK 4-6 (SOFT FOODS, PHASE 3) (30)

Contents

Chocolate And Banana Pudding

Servings: 4 / Preparation Time: 2 hours/ Cooking Time: 5 minutes

The most perfect and delicious Chocolate and Banana Pudding for your phase 3 journey!

1 cup almond milk

1 cup chocolate, melted

4 bananas, peeled and sliced

½ cup condensed almond milk

2 tablespoons butter

2 tablespoons cocoa powder

1 cup coconut cream

- Take a saucepan and add butter and let it cook until reduced to half, add condensed almond milk, chocolate, cocoa powder, and stir.
- Add half of the chocolate pudding into a large dish and place banana slices evenly.
- Pour remaining chocolate on top and freeze for 2 hours.
- Top with whipped cream and enjoy!

Per Serving: Calories: 187; Total Fat: 4g; Saturated Fat: 0g; Protein: 4g; Carbs: 34g; Fiber: 10g

Carrot Pudding

Servings: 4 / Preparation Time: 10 minutes/ Cooking Time: 15 minutes

If you want to avoid chocolate and walk the veggie path, this delicious Carrot Pudding is the way to go!

2/3 cup carrot puree

1 teaspoon vanilla paste

1 teaspoon lemon zest

4 cups of coconut milk

Cornstarch (a mixture of 2 tablespoons cornstarch and 4 tablespoons water)

1 whole egg

- Add carrot and milk in a saucepan and place it over low heat, cover and cook until tiny bubbles appear.
- Whisk egg, cornstarch slurry, lemon zest in a bowl and add into the pan in a steady stream.
- Cover and cook for 15 minutes more.
- Divide between dessert bowls and enjoy!

Per Serving: Calories: 159; Total Fat: 10g; Saturated Fat: 2g; Protein: 4g; Carbs: 18g; Fiber: 3g

Fancy Scrambled Eggs

Servings: 4 / Preparation Time: 5 minutes/ Cooking Time: 5-10 minutes

The most traditional Scrambled Eggs recipe for every morning!

4 whole eggs

1/8 teaspoon salt

1/8 teaspoon pepper

2 tablespoons olive oil

2 tablespoons red bell pepper, chopped

1 garlic clove, chopped

1 and ½ teaspoons chives, chopped

- Take a bowl and beat eggs, pepper, and salt.
- Take a large skillet and place it over medium heat, add oil, red bell pepper, garlic and cook for 5 minutes.
- Add egg mixture and chives to skillet.
- Cook and stir over low heat until eggs are cooked.
- Enjoy!

Per Serving: Calories: 199; Total Fat: 15g; Saturated Fat: 2g; Protein: 13g; Carbs: 2g; Fiber: 0g

Yogurt Crème Brulee Custard

Servings: 4 / Preparation Time: 10 minutes/ Cooking Time: nil

Despite the misconception of Crème Brulee being extremely difficult, this simple recipe will basically make things easier and easy to consume!

2 cups thick Greek yogurt   1 cup strawberries puree

- Take a bowl and add strawberries puree and yogurt.
- Divide the mixture between four ramekins.
- Serve and enjoy!

Per Serving: Calories: 357; Total Fat: 27g; Saturated Fat: 4g; Protein: 6g; Carbs: 22g; Fiber: 4g

BBQ'd Baked Beans

Servings: 4 / Preparation Time: 10 minutes/ Cooking Time: 60 minutes

You've heard of BBQ meat, but have you heard of BBQ baked beans? If not, then this is your chance to go with it!

1 yellow onion, chopped

5 garlic cloves, minced

¼ pound potatoes, peeled and diced

1 pound into

6 cups of water

1 cup BBQ sauce

2 tablespoons spicy brown mustard

2 tablespoons adobo sauce

Splash of Guinness

2 teaspoons salt

1 teaspoon pepper

- Wash beans thoroughly and soak overnight.
- Set your Dutch oven to pre-heat on top of the stove and add potatoes to the oven, let them brown.
- Add onions and Sauté until tender.
- Keep Sautéing and add garlic, cook for 1 minute.
- Pour beans, water, and cover, cook on low for 60 minutes until beans are tender.
- Add a bit of BBQ sauce, adobo sauce, mustard salt, pepper, and stir.
- Remove cover and let it simmer until sauce thickens and beans are cooked thoroughly.

Per Serving: Calories: 70; Total Fat: 1g; Saturated Fat: 0g; Protein: 3g; Carbs: 14g; Fiber: 3g

Easy Baked Tomatoes

Servings: 5 / Preparation Time: 10 minutes/ Cooking Time: 50 minutes

Hearty whole tomatoes baked to perfection for your guilty pleasure!

¼ cup pine nuts

Greek seasoning as needed

¼ cup low-fat parmesan

Olive oil spray as needed

5-6 whole tomatoes

- Pre-heat your oven to 350 degrees F.
- Slice tomatoes in half lengthwise and transfer to a pan with cut side up.
- Spray tops of tomato with olive oil spray.
- Season with pine nuts, cheese, and Greek seasoning.
- Bake for 50 minutes and serve, enjoy!

Per Serving: Calories: 73; Total Fat: 5g; Saturated Fat: 1g; Protein: 3g; Carbs: 6g; Fiber: 1g

Black Bean Chipotle Hummus

Servings: 4 / Preparation Time: 5 minutes/ Cooking Time: nil

Very soft and tender black bean hummus with a fine heat coming from the chipotle. GO in if you dare.

1 (15 ounces) can, black beans, drained and rinsed

1 lime, juiced

1 chipotle pepper in adobo sauce

1 teaspoon adobo sauce

1 teaspoon garlic, minced

2 teaspoons ground cumin

2 tablespoons extra-virgin olive oil

¼ cup fresh cilantro, chopped

- Take your food processor and add black beans, lime juice, chipotle pepper, adobo sauce, garlic, cumin, olive oil, cilantro and blend on high for 2-3 minutes until smooth.
- Serve and enjoy!

Per Serving: Calories: 52; Total Fat: 2g; Saturated Fat: 1g; Protein: 2g; Carbs: 6g; Fiber: 1g

Finely Crispy Wok Veggies

Servings: 2 / Preparation Time: 10 minutes/ Cooking Time: 20 minutes

Looking for a quick veggie fix? This easy Wok Fried veggie is all you need!

1 medium red bell pepper, cut into strips

1 medium green bell pepper, cut into strips

7-8 pieces baby corn

½ cup button mushrooms, canned

1 cup cauliflower, chopped into bite-sized pieces

1 medium carrot, peeled and cut into strips

1 teaspoon oyster sauce

1 tablespoon olive oil

1 teaspoon salt

- Wash bell peppers and cut them in half.

- Remove seeds and cut into strips.

- Take a large wok pan and heat up olive oil over medium heat, add carrots and cauliflower and cook for 8-10 minutes.

- Add red and green pepper strips, baby corn, button mushrooms, oyster sauce, cook for 5-7 minutes.

- Serve veggies with mashed potatoes and sprinkled turmeric.

- Enjoy!

Per Serving: Calories: 236; Total Fat: 6g; Saturated Fat: 0g; Protein: 9g; Carbs: 46g; Fiber: 8g

Cheesy Tomato Omelet

Servings: 4 / Preparation Time: 5 minutes/ Cooking Time: 5-10 minutes

Yet another fantastic way to start off your day! Cook up a batch of cheesy tomato omelet and energize yourself for the rest of the day!

½ teaspoon butter

1 large whole egg

1 tablespoon milk

Salt and pepper to taste

Garlic powder

1 slice cheddar cheese

1 tablespoon tomato, chopped

- Take a 6-inch non-stick skillet and melt butter over medium heat, coat well.
- Take a small bowl and whisk in egg, milk and pour into skillet.
- Season with garlic, pepper, salt.
- Once the edges of the egg mix begin to cook, lift with spatula and tip skillet so uncooked egg flows underneath.
- Repeat step 3 until top is almost dry. Place cheese slice on top then tomato over half omelet.
- Once cheese begins to melt, fold in half and serve.

Per Serving: Calories: 227; Total Fat: 19g; Saturated Fat: 2g; Protein: 18g; Carbs: 7g; Fiber: 2g

Stuffed Avocado

Servings: 4 / Preparation Time: 15 minutes/ Cooking Time: 20 minutes

Avocados are already extremely versatile! But, if you are not in the mode for the world famous Guacamole, just go in and prepare these stuffed avocados!

2 medium-sized ripe avocado, cut in half

6 large eggs

1 medium tomato, finely chopped

3 tablespoons olive oil

2 tablespoons fresh parsley, chopped

4 tablespoons Greek yogurt

1 tablespoon fresh rosemary, chopped

½ teaspoon salt

¼ teaspoon pepper, ground

- Pre-heat your oven to 350 degrees F.
- Take a small baking dish and grease with oil, keep it on the side.
- Cut avocado in half and scrape out flesh from the center.
- Take a medium bowl and whisk in eggs, tomatoes, parsley, rosemary, salt, and pepper.
- Stir until thoroughly incorporated, spoon mixture into avocado shells.
- Spread stuffed avocado on a baking sheet and bake for 15-20 minutes.
- Remove and top with yogurt, enjoy!

Per Serving: Calories: 385; Total Fat: 35g; Saturated Fat: 5g; Protein: 10g; Carbs: 12g; Fiber: 2g

Best Chocolate Porridge

Servings: 6 / Preparation Time: 1 minute/ Cooking Time: 3 minutes

Yet another breakfast dish to satisfy your early morning cravings.

Small square dark unsweetened chocolate

1 tablespoon low-calorie sweetener

1 tablespoon chocolate protein powder

3 tablespoons porridge oats

1 cup skimmed milk

- Add chocolate, protein powder, milk and oats to a jug.
- Mix well and transfer to microwave container, cook for 2 minutes.
- Stir and cook for 20-30 seconds more.
- Mix in your desired sweetener and spoon mixture into serving bowl.
- Top with couple blackberries and a bit of chopped chocolate.
- Enjoy!

Per Serving: Calories: 328; Total Fat: 8g; Saturated Fat: 1g; Protein: 23g; Carbs: 41g; Fiber: 10g

Chocolate Chia Pudding

Servings: 4 / Preparation Time: 10 minutes + 60 minutes to chill/ Cooking Time: nil

A fine dessert that packs a good amount of fiber and choco flavor.

2 cups unsweetened soy milk

10 drops liquid stevia

¼ cup unsweetened cocoa powder

¼ teaspoon ground cinnamon

¼ teaspoon vanilla extract

½ cup chia seeds

½ cup fresh raspberries, for garnish

- Take a small sized bowl and whisk in soy milk, stevia, cocoa powder, cinnamon, vanilla and mix well until combined.
- Stir in chia seeds.
- Divide the mixture between 4 small dishes.
- Cover and let it chill for 1 hour.
- Once done, garnish with raspberries, enjoy!

Per Serving: Calories: 182; Total Fat: 9g; Saturated Fat: 2g; Protein: 11g; Carbs: 14g; Fiber: 14g

Tender Soft Mexican Chicken Salad

Servings: 5 / Preparation Time: 5 minutes/ Cooking Time: 5 minutes

Awesome Mexican Chicken Salad for any meal of the day!

2 teaspoons juice of jarred salsa

1 teaspoon taco seasoning

1 tablespoon light mayonnaise

1 cup canned chicken, drained

- Add drained chicken in a bowl and take a fork, break chicken into small pieces.
- Add mayonnaise to chicken and combine well, mash chicken into mayonnaise with a fork.
- Add salsa juice and taco seasoning to chicken mix, keep mixing and mash everything well.
- Serve and enjoy!

Per Serving: Calories: 180; Total Fat: 5g; Saturated Fat: 1g; Protein: 21g; Carbs: 10g; Fiber: 2g

Protein Packed Pumpkin Pie Oatmeal

Servings: 5 / Preparation Time: 5 minutes/ Cooking Time: 5 minutes

A pumpkin flavored delicious Oatmeal that will just keep you wanting for more!

1 cup 1% cottage cheese

1 teaspoon Truvia baking blend

Dash of ginger

Dash of cloves

Dash of cinnamon

½ cup canned pumpkin

½ cup old fashioned oats

- Add sweetener, spices, pumpkin, and oats in a microwave proof bowl.
- Cook for 90 seconds on HIGH and stir in cottage cheese.
- Microwave for 60 seconds more.
- Let it stand for a minute and enjoy!

Per Serving: Calories: 205; Total Fat: 3g; Saturated Fat: 0g; Protein: 14g; Carbs: 34g; Fiber: 6g

Delicious Mugastrone

Servings: 2 / Preparation Time: 1 minute/ Cooking Time: 5 minutes

The famous Mugastrone recipe for phase 3 of your journey, enjoy!

Salt and pepper to taste

¼ ounces dry vermicelli

1 and ½ tablespoons frozen mixed vegetables

1 tablespoon cooked borlotti beans

2/3 cup tomato juice

- Add tomato sauce to a glass measuring cup, add pepper, salt, noodles, veggies, and beans. Stir well.

- Transfer to microwave and cook for 2-3 minutes.

- Top with parmesan and enjoy!

Per Serving: Calories: 170; Total Fat: 4g; Saturated Fat: 1g; Protein: 5g; Carbs: 16g; Fiber: 4g

Lemon-Blackberry Frozen Yogurt

Servings: 4 / Preparation Time: 10 minutes/ Cooking Time: nil

Looking for something of your next Dessert? Just whip up this Lemon-Blackberry Yogurt for the delight of your friends and family, and yourself!

4 cups frozen blackberries

½ cup low-fat plain Greek yogurt

1 lemon, juiced

2 teaspoons liquid stevia

Fresh mint leaves, for garnish

- Take your food processor and ad blackberries, yogurt, lemon juice, stevia and blend well until smooth.
- Serve immediately and enjoy with a garnish of fresh mint leaves.

Per Serving: Calories: 68; Total Fat: 0g; Saturated Fat: 0g; Protein: 3g; Carbs: 15g; Fiber: 5g

Creamy Cauliflower Dish

Servings: 5 / Preparation Time: 10 minutes/ Cooking Time: 5 minutes

Fantastic Cauliflower dish, but made extremely creamy and delicious thanks to the addition of buttermilk and butter, awesome!

½ teaspoon pepper

4 teaspoon extra virgin olive oil

½ teaspoon garlic salt

1 teaspoon salted butter

1/3 cup low-fat buttermilk

3 cloves garlic

Large head of cauliflower

- Break your cauliflower into small florets and transfer to a large microwave proof bowl, add garlic and a quarter of water.

- Microwave for 5 minutes until cauliflower is tender.

- Use a garlic press and crush garlic cloves, add to food processor and add to cauliflower.

- Add pepper, garlic salt, butter, two teaspoons olive oil, buttermilk.

- Process well until creamy and smooth.

- Drizzle remaining olive oil on top and enjoy!

Per Serving: Calories: 113; Total Fat: 6g; Saturated Fat: 2g; Protein: 5g; Carbs: 13g; Fiber: 3g

Beetroot And Butterbean Hummus

Servings: 4 / Preparation Time: 5 minutes/ Cooking Time: nil

Yet another Hummus recipe, but this time with Beetroot and Butterbean goes best with a fine selection of sides.

Salt and pepper as needed

1 tablespoon extra-virgin olive oil

2 tablespoons Fat-Free Greek yogurt

Bunch of chives, chopped

1-2 cloves garlic, crushed

14 ounces butterbeans, drained and rinsed

8 ounces cooked beetroot

- Dice beetroot and cut into small cubes.
- Add butterbeans in a food processor and season with salt, pepper, yogurt, oil, chives, and garlic.
- Blitz until the mixture is a nice puree.
- Fold in diced beetroot and blitz gently.
- Serve and enjoy!

Per Serving: Calories: 80; Total Fat: 2g; Saturated Fat: 0g; Protein: 4.2g; Carbs: 10g; Fiber: 0.5g

Raisin And Oats Mug Cakes

Servings: 3 / Preparation Time: 10 minutes/ Cooking Time: 1 minute

The perfect Raisin and Oats Mug Cake for every morning takes very little time to prepare and is bursting with flavor.

1 and ½ tablespoons flour

1 and ½ tablespoons almond milk

½ tablespoon raisins

¼ teaspoon baking powder

1/16 teaspoon salt

½ tablespoons canola oil

1/8 teaspoons baking soda

1/8 teaspoons vanilla extract

1/8 teaspoons hazelnut extract

¾ tablespoons oats

1 teaspoon lemon juice

¼ teaspoon baking powder

- Whisk in all ingredients in a microwave-proof mug and cook on high for 1 minute.
- Let it cool, serve and enjoy!

Per Serving: Calories: 185; Total Fat: 1.7g; Saturated Fat: 1g; Protein: 8g; Carbs: 39g; Fiber: 10g

No-Bake Peanut Butter Protein Bites And Dark Chocolate

Servings: 10 / Preparation Time: 20 minutes + chill time/ Cooking Time: nil

This amazing dessert won't require you to bake it, but just add the ingredients and let it chill, then be ready to go for a feast of a lifetime!

1 cup old fashioned rolled oats	1 tablespoon chia seeds
1 cup vanilla protein powder	1 teaspoon vanilla extract
¾ cup smooth natural peanut butter	¼ cup dark chocolate chips
2 tablespoons ground flaxseed	¾ teaspoons stevia baking blend
1 tablespoon ground flaxseed	1 tablespoon water

- Take a bowl and mix In oats, protein powder, peanut butter, flaxseed, chia seeds, vanilla, chocolate chips, stevia, and water.
- Let it chill for 30 minutes.
- Roll the mixture into 25 balls, eat and enjoy!

Per Serving: Calories: 181; Total Fat: 10g; Saturated Fat: 0g; Protein: 11g; Carbs: 11g; Fiber: 3g

Hearty Overnight Oats

Servings: 4 / Preparation Time: 3 minutes + 12 hours overnight sit / Cooking Time: nil

No fuss, everyday overnight oats. Perfect to give you a boost of fiber.

¾ cup Fat-Free Greek yogurt

2 tablespoons protein powder

1 and ¼ cup semi-skimmed milk

2 tablespoons Chia seeds

1 cup porridge oats

- Add yogurt, protein powder, milk, chia seeds, and oats in a bowl and mix well.
- Spoon mixture into four servings and cover them.
- Let the mixture sit in the fridge overnight.
- Serve by stirring the mixture and topping it with seeds, nuts, and fruits.
- Enjoy!

Per Serving: Calories: 338; Total Fat: 10g; Saturated Fat: 2g; Protein: 22g; Carbs: 34g; Fiber: 9g

Awesome Cheesy Grits

Servings: 4 / Preparation Time: 5 minutes/ Cooking Time: 5-10 minutes

Perfectly Surgery friendly cheesy Grits, that's all you need for a nice snack!

1 cup uncooked grits   ¼ cup half and half

5 whole eggs

1 cup cheddar cheese, shredded

- Prepare your grits according to the packet.

- Take a small bowl and mix in beaten eggs and cheese.

- Once grits are done, stir in 3 tablespoons hot grits into egg mixture.

- Add egg mixture to the cooking grits, whisk in egg mixture into grits until smooth.

- Add half and half, whisk until grits reach your desired consistency.

- Enjoy!

Per Serving: Calories: 304; Total Fat: 10g; Saturated Fat: 2g; Protein: 16g; Carbs: 36g; Fiber: 6g

Pumpkin Porridge

Servings: 3 / Preparation Time: 10 minutes/ Cooking Time: 30 minutes

If you are bored of the normal Porridge, then add pumpkin to the mix! It will completely change how you perceive the taste of a porridge.

1 cup pumpkin, chopped

1 cup fresh arugula, chopped

3 tablespoons almonds, ground

1 teaspoon dry rosemary, chopped

½ teaspoon dry thyme, ground

1 tablespoon olive oil

- Pre-heat your oven to 350 degrees F.

- Peel pumpkin and cut it lengthwise in half. Scrape out seeds and one large wedge.

- Cut into fine chunks and fill up measuring cup, wrap remaining of pumpkin in plastic foil and chill for a while.

- Take a large baking sheet and grease with olive oil, spread pumpkin and sprinkle rosemary and thyme.

- Bake for 30 minutes, remove from oven and let them cool.

- Take a bowl and add arugula, ground almonds, add baked pumpkin and drizzle olive oil.

- Stir well and enjoy!

Per Serving: Calories: 158; Total Fat: 12g; Saturated Fat: 2g; Protein: 5g; Carbs: 12g; Fiber: 3g

Fancy Vegan Porridge

Servings: 2 / Preparation Time: 5 minute/ Cooking Time: 5 minutes

Porridge for the Vegan lovers just digs in!

2 tablespoons coconut flour

3 tablespoons flaxseed meal

2 tablespoons protein powder

1 and ½ cups unsweetened almond milk

Powdered Erythritol

- Take a bowl and add flaxseed, coconut flour, protein powder.
- Take a saucepan and place it over medium heat, add almond milk and cook until the mixture starts to thicken.
- Stir in a preferred portion of sweetener and serve with your desired topping.
- Enjoy!

Per Serving: Calories: 112; Total Fat: 5g; Saturated Fat: 1g; Protein: 4g; Carbs: 11g; Fiber: 4g

Strawberry Orange Salad

Servings: 4 / Preparation Time: 10 minutes/ Cooking Time: nil

A platter of Strawberry and Orange that will not only fill up your tummy but give you a health boost too!

1 cup fresh strawberries, chopped

1 medium-sized orange, chopped

½ cup fresh cranberries

1 cup romaine lettuce, chopped

3 tablespoons lemon juice, squeezed

¼ teaspoon cinnamon, ground

- Wash strawberries thoroughly and cut into bite-sized portions.
- Add cranberries to a colander and wash under cold water, drain them.
- Wash lettuce thoroughly and roughly chop, peel orange and divide into wedges.
- Cut each wedge in half and keep it on the side.
- Take a small bowl and add lemon juice, cinnamon, stir well.
- Add strawberries, cranberries lettuce in salad bowl.
- Drizzle dressing and serve, enjoy!

Per Serving: Calories: 79; Total Fat: 0.5g; Saturated Fat: 0g; Protein: 1.4g; Carbs: 17g; Fiber: 2g

Delicious Jelly And Buttery Pancakes

Servings: 5 / Preparation Time: 5 minutes/ Cooking Time: 10 minutes

The perfect way to start your day! A delicious platter of spiced up scrambled eggs!

An assorted collection of frozen mixed berries

4 egg whites

2 tablespoons powdered peanuts

½ cup instant oatmeal

½ cup low-fat cottage cheese

- Add egg whites, powdered peanut, oatmeal, and cottage cheese into a blender.
- Mix until you have a nice and smooth batter.
- Pour mixture into and fold in berry mix.
- Spray oil and divide the batter into portions.
- Pour batter and cook for 2-3 minutes each side until golden brown.
- Enjoy!

Per Serving: Calories: 90; Total Fat: 1.5g; Saturated Fat: 0g; Protein: 10g; Carbs: 9g; Fiber: 1g

Chocolate Brownies With Almond Butter

Servings: 6 / Preparation Time: 5 minutes/ Cooking Time: 25 minutes

Heartiest chocolate brownie out there! The added Almond Butter just sweetens the deal even more!

½ cup of cocoa powder

1 tablespoon ground flaxseed

½ teaspoon ground instant coffee

¼ teaspoon baking soda

½ cup almond butter

¼ cups melted coconut oil

2 large eggs

1 teaspoon vanilla extra

½ cup agave nectar

- Pre-heat your oven to 325 degrees F.

- Take an 8 x 8-inch glass baking dish and grease it.

- Take a food processor and add cocoa powder, flaxseed, instant coffee, baking soda, almond butter, coconut oil, eggs, vanilla, agave nectar and process in high until smooth.

- Pour the batter into baking dish.

- Bake for 25 minutes, until a toothpick, comes out clean from the middle.

- Let it cool for 10 minutes and cut into squares.

- Enjoy!

Per Serving: Calories: 124; Total Fat: 9g; Saturated Fat: 3g; Protein: 3g; Carbs: 11g; Fiber: 2g

Chunky Mediterranean Tomato Soup

Servings: 4 / Preparation Time: 5 minutes/ Cooking Time: 5-10 minutes

Mediterranean Soup with chunked up veggies, it doesn't get better than this!

3 and ½ cups grilled vegetable mix, frozen

2 tablespoons garlic, chopped

Fresh basil leaves

3 and ½ cups tomato, chopped

1 low-salt veggie stock cube

½ cup ricotta

- Take a pan and place it over medium heat, add vegetables and garlic, cook until veggies are tender.

- Add basil, tomatoes, stock cube and two cans water.

- Puree the mixture to a chunky mixture using an immersion blender.

- Enjoy!

Per Serving: Calories: 212; Total Fat: 10g; Saturated Fat: 0g; Protein: 11g; Carbs: 24g; Fiber: 2g

Frozen Raspberry Cream

Servings: 2 / Preparation Time: 5 minutes/ Cooking Time: nil

Amazing Frozen Raspberry Cream, looking for a dessert? Just go for this one! The cherry extract on the recipe is literally the "Cherry On Top"

1 cup almond cream

1 cup fresh raspberry

¼ cup skim milk

1 tablespoon cherry extract

2 tablespoons honey, raw

- Wash raspberries using a large colander and drain them, keep them on the side.

- Take a large bowl and add all the ingredients, beat using a fork.

- Pour mixture into paper cups and freeze for 30 minutes.

- Garnish with nuts and add a teaspoon of lemon juice for extra nutrients, enjoy!

Per Serving: Calories: 140; Total Fat: 0g; Saturated Fat: 0g; Protein: 5g; Carbs: 34g; Fiber: 4g

Braised Swiss Chard

Servings: 2 / Preparation Time: 5 minutes/ Cooking Time: 25 minutes

Braise them Swiss Chard real good for an excellent almost char like flavor in your chard, goes amazing with the addition of potatoes and spices.

1 pound Swiss chard, torn

2 medium-sized potatoes, peeled and finely chopped

3 tablespoons extra-virgin olive oil

1 small onion, chopped

2 garlic cloves, finely chopped

1 teaspoon salt

¼ teaspoon pepper, ground

- Wash Swiss chard thoroughly under cold running water and tear them.
- Add Swiss Chard in a large heavy-bottomed pot and add enough water to cover it, bring to a boil and cook for 3 minutes.
- Drain and keep on the side.
- Pre-heat oil in large skillet over medium-high heat and add onions and garlic, stir cook for 3-4 minutes.
- Add potatoes and 1 cup water bring to a boil, lower heat to low and cook for 15 minutes.
- Add Swiss chard and season with salt and pepper. Cook for 2 and remove heat.
- Serve and enjoy!

Per Serving: Calories: 260; Total Fat: 14g; Saturated Fat: 2g; Protein: 5g; Carbs: 30g; Fiber: 6g

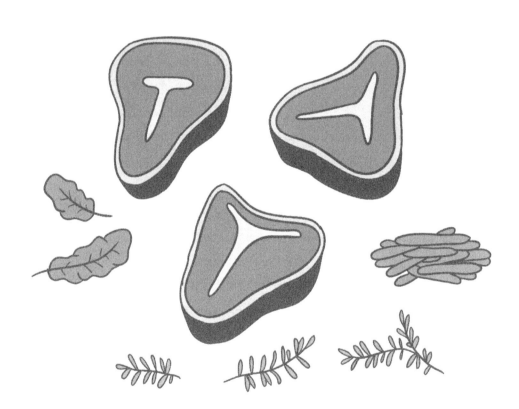

CHAPTER 4: WEEK 7-8 (GENERAL DIET, PHASE 4) (30)

Contents

Hearty Cinnamon Oatmeal

Servings: 10 / Preparation Time: 5 minutes/ Cooking Time: 7-8 hours

Fancy early morning Cinnamon flavored Oatmeal, what more could you ask for ?

8 cups of water

2 cups steel-cut oats

2 teaspoons ground cinnamon

1 teaspoon ground nutmeg

For extra protein:

½ cup low-fat milk

2 tablespoons unflavored vanilla protein powder

2 tablespoons egg white powder

2 tablespoons powdered peanut butter

Extra add-ins:

½ cup fresh berries

½ apple, peeled and sliced

¼ cup pumpkin puree

- Add water, oats, cinnamon, and nutmegs to your Slow Cooker.
- Cover and cook on LOW for 7-8 hours.
- Choose one of your desired protein and add-ins and mix it in before serving.
- Enjoy!

Per Serving: Calories: 136; Total Fat: 2g; Saturated Fat: 1g; Protein: 6g; Carbs: 23g; Fiber: 4g

Cheesy Broccoli Soup

Servings: 4 / Preparation Time: 10 minutes/ Cooking Time: 20 minutes

If you are looking for a cheesy and creamy soup that still packs a healthy punch, this is the one that you need!

1 tablespoon extra-virgin olive oil

1 medium onion, chopped

1 tablespoon garlic, minced

2 cups carrots, grated

¼ teaspoon ground nutmeg

¼ cup whole wheat pastry flour

2 cups low sodium vegetable broth

2 cups non-fat milk

½ cup fat-free half and half

3 cups broccoli florets

2 cups extra sharp cheddar cheese, shredded

- Take a stock pot and heat up olive oil over medium heat, add onion and garlic and Saute for 1 minute.

- Add carrots, and stir cook for 2-3 minutes until tender.

- Add nutmeg, flour and cook stirring for 2-3 minutes until browned.

- Add broth and milk and whisk well, add half and half and mix well.

- Stir in broccoli florets and bring to a boil, lower heat to low and simmer for 10 minutes.

- Stir in cheddar cheese until melted, top with more cheese and enjoy!

Per Serving: Calories: 193; Total Fat: 9g; Saturated Fat: 0g; Protein: 12g; Carbs: 17g; Fiber: 5g

Kiwi Banana Oatmeal

Servings: 3 / Preparation Time: 15-20 minutes/ Cooking Time: 5 minutes

Delicious Banana and Kiwi flavored oatmeal for every warm morning, a refreshing delight to start your day with!

2 large kiwis, peeled

1 large banana

1 cup rolled oats

1 cup milk

1 tablespoon chia seeds

¼ cup raisins

1 tablespoon raisins

1 tablespoon honey, raw

1 tablespoon almonds, roughly chopped

- Peel kiwis and banana, cut into thin slices and keep it on the side.
- Heat up milk in a deep pot and over medium-high temperature, make sure to not bring it to a boil. Remove from heat and stir in rolled oats.
- Stir well until incorporated, soak for 15 minutes.
- Stir in raisins, honey, chia seeds. Top with kiwi, banana and sprinkle almonds.
- Enjoy!

Per Serving: Calories: 330; Total Fat: 7g; Saturated Fat: 1g; Protein: 10g; Carbs: 60g; Fiber: 10g

High-Protein Pancake

Servings: 4 / Preparation Time: 5 minutes/ Cooking Time: 5 minutes

Morning Pancakes packed to the brim with a buck load of protein!

3 whole eggs

1 cup low-fat cottage cheese

1/3 cup whole-wheat pastry flour

1 and ½ tablespoons coconut oil, melted

Non-stick cooking spray

- Take a large bowl and whisk in eggs.

- Whisk in cottage cheese, flour, coconut oil until gently combined.

- Take a large skillet and place it over medium heat, lightly coat with cooking spray.

- Use a measuring cup and pour ½ cup of batter into the skillet, cook for a 2-3 minute until bubbles appear all across the surface.

- Flip pancake and cook for 1-2 minutes more until both sides are golden brown.

- Serve and enjoy!

Per Serving: Calories: 182; Total Fat: 10g; Saturated Fat: 2g; Protein: 12g; Carbs: 10g; Fiber: 4g

Hardboiled Eggs And Avocado Toast

Servings: 4 / Preparation Time: 5 minutes/ Cooking Time: 20 minutes

The simplest breakfast that you can conjure up, avocado on a toast alongside hardboiled eggs. The perfect balance.

4 whole eggs

4 slices sprouted whole wheat bread

1 medium avocado

1 teaspoon hot sauce

Fresh ground pepper

- Take a large pot and bring it to a rapid boil on high heat.

- Add eggs to boiling water using and spoon and let them boil for 10 minutes.

- Transfer eggs from boiling water to a strainer and run under cold water ,peel and slice them into fourths.

- Toast your bread.

- Mash avocado with a fork in a small sized bowl and mix in hot sauce.

- Spread avocado mash evenly across each toast and top with 4 egg slices. Season with pepper and enjoy!

Per Serving: Calories: 191; Total Fat: 10g; Saturated Fat: 2g; Protein: 10g; Carbs: 15g; Fiber: 3g

Herbed Crusted Salmon

Servings: 4 / Preparation Time: 10 minutes/ Cooking Time: 30 minutes

Easy to prepared salmon, with a fine herb crust. Once you get past its crunchy exterior, it will literally melt in your mouth.

2 (4 ounces) salmon fillets

2 teaspoons garlic, minced

1 tablespoon dried parsley

½ teaspoon dried thyme

2 teaspoons freshly squeezed lemon

4 tablespoons Parmigiano-Reggiano cheese, grated

- Pre-heat your oven to 425 degrees F.

- Line a rimmed baking sheet with parchment paper.

- Add salmon skin, skin sized own on a baking sheet and cover with the second piece of parchment paper. Bake for 10 minutes.

- Take a bowl and mix in garlic, parsley, thyme, lemon juice, cheese.

- Discard parchment paper covering salmon and use a pastry brush to cover the fillets with herb-cheese mixture.

- Bake for 5 minutes (uncovered)

- Salmon is done once the fish flakes easily with a fork.

Per Serving: Calories: 197; Total Fat: 10g; Saturated Fat: 2g; Protein: 27g; Carbs: 9g; Fiber: 2g

Simple Jerked Chicken With Mango Salsa

Servings: 4 / Preparation Time: 15 minutes + 30 minutes marinade time/ Cooking Time: 15 minutes

A spicy jerked chicken that will satisfy any spice lover! The Mango Salsa will just even the odds here.

2 tablespoons extra virgin olive oil

1 lime, juiced

1 tablespoon garlic, minced

1 teaspoon ginger, ground

½ teaspoon dried thyme

½ teaspoon cinnamon

½ teaspoon ground allspice

½ teaspoon ground nutmeg

¼ teaspoon cayenne pepper

¼ teaspoon ground cloves

1 teaspoon fresh ground black pepper

4 boneless, skinless chicken breasts

1 cup Mango Salsa

- Take a gallon sized zip bag and add olive oil, garlic, lime juice, ginger, thyme, allspice, cinnamon, nutmeg, cloves, cayenne, black pepper.

- Seal and mix to prepare the marinade.

- Add breast to the marinade and tightly seal the bag, shake well to coat the chicken.

- Let it chill for 30 minutes.

- Pre-heat your grill to medium-high heat and add chicken on the grill, discard marinade.

- Cook for 6 minutes on each side until the middle is no longer pink and internal temperature reaches 165 degrees F.

- Let the chicken sit for 5 minutes and slice, enjoy!

Per Serving: Calories: 206; Total Fat: 9g; Saturated Fat: 1g; Protein: 25g; Carbs: 11g; Fiber: 1g

Baked Zucchini Fries

Servings: 4 / Preparation Time: 15 minutes/ Cooking Time: 30 minutes

Zucchini fries are pretty much fan favorite amongst veggie lovers, baking them takes things to another level!

3 large zucchini

2 large eggs

1 cup whole wheat bread crumbs

¼ cup shredded Parmigiano-Reggiano cheese

1 teaspoon garlic powder

1 teaspoon onion powder

- Pre-heat your oven to 425 degrees F.

- Line a large rimmed baking sheet with aluminum foil and halve the zucchini lengthwise.

- Slice each piece into fries with ½ inch diameter.

- Take a small bowl and crack in eggs and beat lightly, take a medium and add bread crumbs, cheese, garlic powder, onion powder.

- Dip each zucchini strip into the egg, roll it into bread crumb mixture and transfer to baking sheet.

- Roast for 30 minutes, stirring fries halfway through, zucchini fries are done once they are brown and crispy.

- Enjoy!

Per Serving: Calories: 89; Total Fat: 3g; Saturated Fat: 2g; Protein: 5g; Carbs: 10g; Fiber: 3g

Lemon And Parsley Crab Cakes

Servings: 4 / Preparation Time: 15 minutes/ Cooking Time: 10 minutes

Let's deviate a little bit from the normal affair and try making some crabs shall we? This simple recipe will give you the best Crab Cakes possible.

3 tablespoons whole wheat bread crumbs

1 egg, lightly beaten

½ teaspoon Dijon mustard

1 and ½ tablespoons olive oil based mayonnaise

¼ teaspoon ground cayenne pepper

2 teaspoons fresh parsley, chopped

Juice of ½ lemons

2 (6 ounces) cans lump crabmeat, drained and cartilage removed

- Take a medium bowl and mix in bread crumbs, egg, mustard, mayonnaise, cayenne pepper, parsley, lemon juice.
- Gently fold in lump crabmeat.
- Use ¼ cup measuring cup and shape mixture into 4 patties.
- Transfer patties to fridge and let it sit for 30 minutes.
- Pre-heat your oven to 500 degrees F. While crab cakes rest in fridge and coat baking sheet with cooking spray.
- Transfer crab cakes on baking sheet and bake for 10 minutes.
- Enjoy!

Per Serving: Calories: 148; Total Fat: 4g; Saturated Fat: 0g; Protein: 21g; Carbs: 5g; Fiber: 1g

Pork, White Bean And Spinach Soup

Servings: 4 / Preparation Time: 10 minutes/ Cooking Time: 50 minutes

A very meaty and porky soup that will leave you licking the bowl until the end.

1 teaspoon extra virgin olive oil

1 medium onion, chopped

2 (4 ounces) boneless pork chops, cut into 1-inch cubes

1 (14 and ½ ounces) can, diced tomatoes

3 cups low-sodium chicken broth

½ teaspoon dried thyme

¼ teaspoon crushed red pepper flakes 1 1 can (15 ounces) great northern beans, drained

8 ounces fresh spinach leaves

- Take a large soup pot and place it over medium heat, add olive oil and let it heat up.

- Add onion, Saute for 2-3 minutes, add pork and brown for 4-5 minutes each side.

- Mix in tomatoes, broth, thyme, red pepper flakes, and beans.

- Bring the mix to a boil and lower down heat to low, simmer for 30 minutes (covered)

- Add spinach and stir well for 5 minutes, serve and enjoy!

Per Serving: Calories: 156; Total Fat: 4g; Saturated Fat: 2g; Protein: 17g; Carbs: 17g; Fiber: 4g

Southwestern Scrambled Egg Burritos

Servings: 4 / Preparation Time: 5 minutes/ Cooking Time: 20 minutes

We have already covered scrambled eggs! Now it's time to teach you how to make scrambled egg burritos! Sound's interesting right? It'll be even awesome once you taste it.

12 whole eggs

¼ cup low-fat milk

1 teaspoon extra virgin olive oil

½ onion, chopped

1 red bell pepper, diced

1 green bell pepper, diced

1 (15 ounces) can black beans, drained and rinsed

8 (7-8 inches) whole wheat tortilla

1 cup salsa for serving

- Take a large bowl and whisk in eggs and milk, keep it on the side.
- Take a large skillet and place it over medium-high heat, heat olive oil and add onions and bell pepper.
- Saute for 2-3 minutes until tender.
- Add beans and stir well to combine.
- Add egg mixture and lower down heat to medium-low, stir gently using a rubber spatula. Cook for 5 minutes until eggs are fluffy and cooked.
- Divide scrambled egg mixture among tortillas and fold bottom end of tortilla, fold in the sides and roll.
- Serve and enjoy!

Per Serving: Calories: 250; Total Fat: 10g; Saturated Fat: 2g; Protein: 19g; Carbs: 28g; Fiber: 10g

Roasted Root Vegetables

Servings: 4 / Preparation Time: 5 minutes/ Cooking Time: 45 minutes

An assorted selection of assorted root vegetables roasted to perfection! A very healthy platter, yours for the taking.

2 medium red beets, peeled

2 large parsnips

2 large carrots, peeled

1 medium butternut squash, peeled and seeded

1 medium red onion

2 tablespoons extra virgin olive oil

4 teaspoons garlic, minced

2 teaspoons dried thyme

- Pre-heat your oven to 425 degrees F.
- Spray a large rimmed baking sheet with cooking spray.
- Roughly chop beets, parsnips, carrots, butternut squash into 1-inch pieces.
- Cut onion into half and cut each half into large chunks.
- Arrange veggies in single, even layer on your baking sheet.
- Sprinkle olive oil, garlic, and thyme.
- Spoon mix to vegetables and coat well with the seasoning.
- Roast for 45 minutes, making sure to stir veggies after every 15 minutes.
- Serve and enjoy!

Per Serving: Calories: 68; Total Fat: 3g; Saturated Fat: 1g; Protein: 1g; Carbs: 5g; Fiber: 1g

Tomato, Cucumber and Basil Salad

Servings: 4 / Preparation Time: 15 minutes + chill time/ Cooking Time: nil

A Salad made from an assorted selection of Basil, Cucumber and Tomato. It will essentially melt your heart.

1 large cucumber, seeded and sliced

4 medium tomatoes, quartered

1 medium red onion, thinly sliced

½ cup fresh basil, chopped

3 tablespoons red wine vinegar

1 tablespoon extra-virgin olive oil

½ teaspoon Dijon mustard

½ teaspoon fresh ground pepper

- Take a medium sized bowl and mix in cucumber, tomatoes, red onion, and basil.
- Take a small bowl and whisk in vinegar, olive oil, mustard, and pepper.
- Pour dressing over veggies and gently stir.
- Cover and chill for 30 minutes.
- Serve and enjoy!

Per Serving: Calories: 72; Total Fat: 4g; Saturated Fat: 2g; Protein: 1g; Carbs: 8g; Fiber: 2g

Slowly Roasted Pesto Salmon

Servings: 4 / Preparation Time: 5 minutes/ Cooking Time: 20 minutes

Perfectly roasted salmon with delicious basil pesto, make this up if you are in for a quick meal.

4 (6 ounces) salmon fillets

4 tablespoons basil pesto

1 teaspoon extra-virgin olive oil

- Pre-heat your oven to 275 degrees F.
- Line a rimmed baking sheet with foil and brush with olive oil.
- Transfer salmon fillets skin-side down on a baking sheet and spread 1 tablespoon pesto on each fillet.
- Roast for 20 minutes.
- Serve and enjoy!

Per Serving: Calories: 182; Total Fat: 10g; Saturated Fat: 2g; Protein: 20g; Carbs: 1g; Fiber: 2g

Chicken Cordon Bleu

Servings: 4 / Preparation Time: 15 minutes/ Cooking Time: 30 minutes

The greatest Chicken and easy Chicken Cordon Bleu for your Gastric Sleeve Surgery diet, it will bring your whole family together.

6 boneless, skinless chicken breasts, thinly sliced

6 slices lean deli ham

6 slices reduced-fat Swiss cheese, halved

2 large eggs

1 tablespoon water

½ cup whole wheat bread crumbs

2 tablespoons Parmigiano-Reggiano cheese

- Pre-heat your oven to 450 degrees F.
- Spray a baking sheet with cooking spray, pound chicken breasts to ¼ inch thickness.
- Layer 1 slice ham and 1 slice (2 halves) cheese on each chicken breast.
- Roll chicken and transfer them to the baking sheet (seam side down).
- Take a small bowl and add whisk in eggs, take another bowl and mix in bread crumbs and cheese.
- Use a pastry brush and lightly brush each chicken roll with egg wash. Sprinkle bread crumbs all over.
- Bake for 30 minutes until the top is lightly browned.
- Enjoy!

Per Serving: Calories: 174; Total Fat: 7g; Saturated Fat: 1g; Protein: 24g; Carbs: 3g; Fiber: 0g

Creamy Chicken Soup And Cauliflower

Servings: 4 / Preparation Time: 15 minutes/ Cooking Time: 40 minutes

Very creamy cauliflower soup with cooked chicken tossed in, a very warm and hearty delight.

1 teaspoon garlic, minced

1 teaspoon extra virgin olive oil

½ yellow onion, diced

1 carrot, diced

1 celery stalk, diced

1 and ½ pounds cooked chicken breast, diced

2 cups low sodium chicken broth

2 cups of water

1 teaspoon fresh ground black pepper

1 teaspoon dried thyme

2 and ½ cups fresh cauliflower florets

1 cup fresh spinach, chopped

2 cups nonfat milk

- Place large soup over medium-high heat and add garlic in olive oil, Sauté for 1 minute.

- Add onion, carrot, celery, Sauté for 3-5 minutes.

- Add chicken breast, broth, water, pepper, thyme, cauliflower and simmer over low-medium heat, cover and cook for 30 minutes.

- Add fresh spinach and stir for 5 minutes.

- Stir in milk and serve, enjoy!

Per Serving: Calories: 164; Total Fat: 3g; Saturated Fat: 0g; Protein: 25g; Carbs: 5g; Fiber: 1g

Mother's Official Sloppy Joes

Servings: 4 / Preparation Time: 10 minutes/ Cooking Time: 30 minutes

Sloppy Joe's are absolutely a fan favorite when backyard party dish, this recipe will teach you how to make them in a matter of minutes.

1 and ½ pound supreme lean ground beef

1 cup onion, chopped

1 cup celery, chopped

1 can (8 ounces) tomato sauce

1/3 cup catsup

2 tablespoons white vinegar

2 tablespoons Worcestershire sauce

2 tablespoons Dijon mustard

1 tablespoon brown sugar

- Take a large skillet and grease with cooking spray, place it over medium heat.

- Add beef and brown for 10 minutes.

- Drain any grease.

- Mix in onion, celery and cook for 2-3 minutes more.

- Stir in tomato sauce, catsup, Worcestershire sauce, mustard, brown sugar, vinegar and bring the whole liquid to a simmer, cook on low for 15 minutes.

- Spoon a ¾ cup of sloppy Joe mix onto each plate, serve and enjoy!

Per Serving: Calories: 269; Total Fat: 5g; Saturated Fat: 2g; Protein: 24g; Carbs: 32g; Fiber: 7g

Cauliflower Rice

Servings: 4 / Preparation Time: 5 minutes/ Cooking Time: 5 minutes

An excellent low-carb alternative to traditional rice, this should help you boost up your weight loss even more.

1 cauliflower head

1 teaspoon extra virgin oil

- Prepare your cauliflower head by removing the stems and leaves, cut into four large sections.
- Add cauliflower to food processor and pulse until it breaks down to a rice-sized texture.
- Transfer rice cauliflower to plate.
- Take a small skillet and place it over medium heat, add olive oil and once the oil is hot, add cauliflower and Sauté for 5-6 minutes.
- Enjoy!

Per Serving: Calories: 12; Total Fat: 0g; Saturated Fat: 0g; Protein: 1g; Carbs: 2g; Fiber: 1g

Barley And Mushroom Risotto

Servings: 4 / Preparation Time: 5 minutes/ Cooking Time: 55 minutes

The fanciest mushroom and barley risotto out there! This is not only healthy but extremely delicious.

1 tablespoon extra-virgin olive oil

1 teaspoon garlic, minced

2 leeks, ends removed and finely chopped, both white and green parts

4 cups mushrooms, sliced

2 teaspoons dried thyme

½ cup pearl barley

½ cup dry white wine

1 and ½ cups low –sodium vegetable broth

1 cup of water

3 cups fresh spinach leaves

- Take a large skillet and place it over medium heat, add olive oil and Sauté garlic for 1 minute.

- Add leeks and Sauté for 2-3 minutes more.

- Add mushrooms and cook for 4 minutes.

- Stir in thyme and barley and cook for 2 minutes more.

- Add wine and stir and simmer over low heat for 5 minutes.

- Add broth and water and cover skillet, simmer for 40 minutes, making sure to stir properly.

- Gently stir in spinach and mix until spinach wilts.

- Enjoy!

Per Serving: Calories: 104; Total Fat: 3g; Saturated Fat: 2g; Protein: 3g; Carbs: 16g; Fiber: 3g

Cheesy Cauliflower Casserole

Servings: 4 / Preparation Time: 10 minutes/ Cooking Time: 55 minutes

Simple and efficient Cauliflower Casserole dish, your neighbors will fall in love with this easy to make the dish!

1 head cauliflower, cut into florets

1 cup low-fat cottage cheese

1 cup low-fat plain Greek yogurt

½ teaspoon Dijon mustard

¼ teaspoon garlic powder

2 ounces (1/2 cup) shredded aged white cheddar cheese

2 ounces (1/2 cup) shredded mild cheddar cheese

- Pre-heat your oven to 350 degrees F.
- Take a medium-sized pot and fill with water $1/3^{rd}$, place steamer basket inside and bring water to a boil over high heat.
- Add cauliflower to the steamer basket, cover pot, and lower heat and bring to a gentle boil and steam cauliflower for 10-15 minutes.
- Steam cauliflower with 2 tablespoons water in microwave on high for 4 minutes.
- Once the cauliflower is steamed, take a medium bowl and add cottage cheese, yogurt, mustard, garlic powder.
- Drain cauliflower in a large colander and gently mash with potato masher, drain out excess water.
- Stir in cauliflower pieces into cottage cheese mixture and mix well.
- Transfer cauliflower mix to an 8 x 8-inch baking dish, bake for 30 minutes.
- Enjoy!

Per Serving: Calories: 147; Total Fat: 7g; Saturated Fat: 2g; Protein: 13g; Carbs: 8g; Fiber: 2g

Yogurt Marinade With Salmon

Servings: 6 / Preparation Time: 65 minutes/ Cooking Time: 30 minutes

An exquisite Salmon Dish with tints of yogurt as its marinade, it'll blow your socks off!

1 pound fresh salmon, cut into bite-sized pieces

1 cup sour cream

1 cup Greek yogurt

3 garlic cloves, crushed

2 large eggs

½ teaspoon salt

1 tablespoon dry parsley

2 tablespoon extra-virgin olive oil

- Pre-heat your oven to 350 degrees F.

- Add sour cream, Greek yogurt, eggs, garlic, salt and dry parsley in a bowl.

- Add salmon slices in the marinade and cover, let it sit for 60 minutes.

- Transfer salmon slices in small baking dish and transfer to oven, bake for 30 minutes.

- Remove from oven and drizzle rest of the marinade on top.

- Serve salmon with steamed asparagus and enjoy!

Per Serving: Calories: 330; Total Fat: 7g; Saturated Fat: 1g; Protein: 10g; Carbs: 60g; Fiber: 10g

Baked Cod With Fennel And Kalamata Olives

Servings: 4 / Preparation Time: 10 minutes/ Cooking Time: 35 minutes

If you are in a rush, this easy baked Cod and Fennel dish should help you satisfy your appetite. The addition of Kalamata Olives will only help you to elevate the flavor.

2 teaspoons extra-virgin olive oil

1 fennel bulb, sliced paper thin

¼ cup dry white wine

1/8 cup fresh squeezed orange juice

1 teaspoon fresh ground black pepper

4 (4 ounces) cod fillets

4 slices fresh orange, with rind

½ cup Kalamata olives pitted

2 bay leaves

- Pre-heat your oven to 400 degrees F.

- Take a large Dutch oven and place it over medium heat, add olive oil and let it heat up.

- Add fennel and cook for 8-10 minutes.

- Add wine and bring to a simmer and cook for 1-2 minutes, stir in orange juice, pepper and simmer for 2 minutes.

- Remove skillet from heat and arrange the cod on top of fennel mixture, add orange slices over fillets.

- Position olives and bay leaves around fish.

- Roast for 20 minutes, until internal temperature reaches 145 degrees F.

- Enjoy!

Per Serving: Calories: 186; Total Fat: 5g; Saturated Fat: 2g; Protein: 21g; Carbs: 8g; Fiber: 2g

Creamy Beef Stroganoff And Mushrooms

Servings: 4 / Preparation Time: 10 minutes/ Cooking Time: 20 minutes

The Awesome-est Beef Stroganoff you could imagine cooking up at home. With a buck load of ingredients and add mushrooms, this is the perfect dish for lunch or dinner.

1 and ½ pounds extra-lean beef sirloin, cut into ½ inch strips

1 teaspoon extra virgin olive oil

1 medium onion, chopped

½ pound mushrooms, sliced

2 tablespoon whole wheat flour

1 cup low-sodium beef broth

1 cup of water

1 teaspoon Worcestershire sauce

½ teaspoon dried thyme

½ teaspoon dried dill

½ cup low fat plain Greek yogurt

2 tablespoons fresh parsley, chopped

- Coat medium pan with cooking spray and place it over medium-high heat.

- Add beef and cook for 5 minutes until browned.

- Transfer to a bowl.

- Add olive oil to the same pan and let it heat up over medium-high heat, add onion and cook for 1-2 minutes.

- Add mushrooms and cook for 3 minutes. Mix in flour and stir to coat onion and mushrooms, stir in broth, water, Worcestershire sauce, thyme drill and bring the whole mixture to boil.

- Cover pan and cook for 10 minutes.

- Stir in yogurt, mix in beef and serve with a garnish of parsley.

- Enjoy!

Per Serving: Calories: 351; Total Fat: 9g; Saturated Fat: 2g; Protein: 31g; Carbs: 30g; Fiber: 5g

Delicious Ranch Seasoned Crispy Chicken Tenders

Servings: 4 / Preparation Time: 10 minutes/ Cooking Time: 20 minutes

Missing KFC styled chicken tenders? Try out this fantastically seasoned chicken tenders. You'll fall in love!

6 chicken tenderloin pieces

2 tablespoons whole wheat pastry flour

1 egg, lightly beaten

½ cup whole wheat bread crumbs

2 tablespoons grated Parmigiano-Reggiano cheese

2 teaspoons dried parsley

¼ teaspoon dried dill

¼ teaspoon onion powder

¼ teaspoon dried basil

1/8 teaspoon fresh ground black pepper

- Pre-heat your oven to 425 degrees F.

- Prepare three small dishes for coating chicken, add flour in one, egg in second and a mixture of breadcrumbs, cheese, parsley, garlic powder, dill, onion powder, basil and pepper in the third bowl.

- Dip tenderloin into flour and shake off any excess, dip chicken in egg and then finally in the breadcrumb mix.

- Bake for 20 minutes until crispy, enjoy!

Per Serving: Calories: 162; Total Fat: 2g; Saturated Fat: 0g; Protein: 25g; Carbs: 8g; Fiber: 1g

Grilled Chicken Wings

Servings: 6 / Preparation Time: 15 minutes/ Cooking Time: 20 minutes

Lovely grilled chicken wings for every occasion! This is very easy and the seasoning on this is completely spot on. You'll love every single bite of it.

1 and ½ pounds frozen chicken wings

Fresh ground black pepper

1 teaspoon garlic powder

1 cup buffalo

- Pre-heat your grill to 350 degrees F.
- Season wings with pepper and garlic powder, grill wings for 15 minutes per side.
- Once they are browned and crispy, toss grilled wings in Buffalo wings sauce and olive oil.
- Enjoy!

Per Serving: Calories: 82; Total Fat: 6g; Saturated Fat: 1g; Protein: 7g; Carbs: 1g; Fiber: 0g

Buffalo Chicken Wrap

Servings: 4 / Preparation Time: 10 minutes/ Cooking Time: nil

Pulled up Buffalo chicken packed inside a fine wrap, what better you to spend your afternoon?

3 cups rotisserie chicken breast

2 cups romaine lettuce, chopped

1 tomato, diced

½ red onion, finely sliced

¼ cup buffalo wing sauce

¼ cup creamy peppercorn ranch dressing

Chopped raw celery as for garnish

5 small whole grain low carb wraps (as Tumaro's)

- Take a large mixing bowl and add chicken, lettuce, tomato, onion, wing sauce, dressing, and celery.
- Add 1 cup of mixture onto each wrap and foil wrap over the salad.
- Use a toothpick to secure the wrap, enjoy!

Per Serving: Calories: 200; Total Fat: 7g; Saturated Fat: 0g; Protein: 28g; Carbs: 14g; Fiber: 3g

Chipotle Shredded Pork

Servings: 8 / Preparation Time: 10 minutes/ Cooking Time: 6 hours 10 minutes

This pork dish is for the spice lovers out there, if you are bored of the ordinary pork dishes, then spice it up with chipotle!

1 (7.5 ounces) can chipotle pepper in adobo sauce

1 and ½ tablespoon apple cider vinegar

1 tablespoon ground cumin

1 tablespoon dried oregano

Juice of 1 lime

2 pounds pork shoulder, trimmed

- Take your blender and puree chipotle pepper, adobo sauce, apple cider vinegar, cumin, oregano, and lime juice.

- Transfer pork shoulder in the slow cooker and pour the sauce all over.

- Cover Slow Cooker and cook for 6 hours on low.

- Shred the pork using forks and enjoy!

Per Serving: Calories: 260; Total Fat: 11g; Saturated Fat: 1g; Protein: 20g; Carbs: 5g; Fiber: 1g

Hearty Apple Crisps

Servings: 5 / Preparation Time: 15 minutes/ Cooking Time: 45 minutes

A very clean and healthy, not to mention chunky, apple crispies recipe! It'll melt your heart.

6 apples, cored, peeled and cut into 1-inch chunks

½ cup of water

3 teaspoons stevia powder

1 tablespoon cornstarch

½ teaspoon ground cinnamon

¼ teaspoon ground nutmeg

½ a lemon, juiced

¾ cup old fashioned oats

¾ cup whole wheat pastry flour

½ cup low-fat plain Greek yogurt

½ cup low-fat plain Greek yogurt

¼ cup coconut oil, melt

- Pre-heat your oven to 350 degrees F.
- Coat an 8 x 8-inch baking dish with cooking spray.
- Add apples, water, 1 and ½ teaspoons of stevia, corn starch, cinnamon, nutmeg, lemon juice in the baking dish and mix well.
- Bake for 20 minutes.
- Take a medium bowl and add oats, flour, 1 and ½ teaspoons stevia, mix in yogurt, coconut oil and stir until all flour is mixed.
- Evenly cover apple mix with the oatmeal and bake for 25 minutes more.
- Serve and enjoy!

Per Serving: Calories: 170; Total Fat: 6g; Saturated Fat: 0g; Protein: 3g; Carbs: 28g; Fiber: 5g

Broccoli Gorgonzola Soup

Servings: 6 / Preparation Time: 10 minutes/ Cooking Time: 2 hours

Even though making a Gorgonzola Soup might sound slightly difficult at first, once you get the hang of it, this dish will simply become your next favorite soup!

10 ounces Gorgonzola cheese, crumbled

1 cup broccoli, finely chopped

1 tablespoon olive oil

½ cup full-fat milk

½ cup vegetable broth

1 tablespoon parsley, finely chopped

½ teaspoon salt

1 tablespoon parsley, finely chopped

½ teaspoon salt

¼ teaspoon black pepper, ground

- Wash your broccoli well under cold water and drain them, chop into bite-sized portions.
- Grease bottom of a deep pot with olive oil and add listed ingredients and 3 cups of water.
- Mix well and cover with lid, cook for 2 hours on low heat.
- Remove heat and sprinkle fresh parsley.
- Serve and enjoy!

Per Serving: Calories: 204; Total Fat: 16g; Saturated Fat: 3g; Protein: 11g; Carbs: 5g; Fiber: 2g

Delicious Vegetable Paella

Servings: 4 / Preparation Time: 10 minutes/ Cooking Time: 3 hours 20 minutes

Easy to make vegetable Paella, the assorted selection of veggies and spices will make your taste buds dance!

½ cup fresh green peas

2 small carrots, finely chopped

1 cup fire-roasted tomatoes

1 cup zucchini, chopped

½ cup celery root, finely chopped

8 saffron threads

1 tablespoon turmeric, ground

1 teaspoon salt

½ teaspoon fresh ground black pepper

2 cups vegetable broth

1 cup long grain rice

- Add all of the listed ingredients in a deep pot (except rice) and stir well.
- Place lid and bring to a boil, lower heat to low and cook for 3 hours until peas are tender.
- Stir in rice and cook for 15-20 minutes more.
- Remove heat and sprinkle parsley, serve warm and enjoy!

Per Serving: Calories: 267; Total Fat: 2g; Saturated Fat: 0g; Protein: 9g; Carbs: 52g; Fiber: 4g

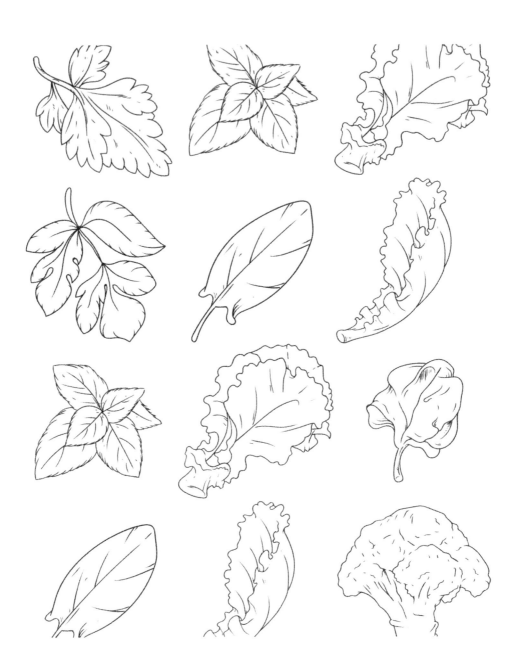

THE "DIRTY DOZEN" AND "CLEAN 15"

Every year, the Environmental Working Group releases a list of the produce with the most pesticide residue (Dirty Dozen) and a list of the ones with the least **chance of having residue (Clean 15). It's based on analysis from the U.S.** Department of Agriculture Pesticide Data Program report.

The Environmental Working Group found that 70% of the 48 types of produce tested had residues of at least one type of pesticide. In total there were 178 different pesticides and pesticide breakdown products. This residue can stay on veggies and fruit even after they are washed and peeled. All pesticides are toxic to humans and consuming them can cause damage to the nervous system, reproductive system, cancer, a weakened immune system, and more. Women who are pregnant can expose their unborn children to toxins through their diet, and continued exposure to pesticides can affect their development.

This info can help you choose the best fruits and veggies, as well as which ones you should always try to buy organic.

The Dirty Dozen

- Strawberries
- Spinach
- Nectarines
- Apples
- Peaches
- Celery
- Grapes
- Pears
- Cherries
- Tomatoes
- Sweet bell peppers
- Potatoes

The Clean 15

- Sweet corn
- Avocados
- Pineapples
- Cabbage
- Onions
- Frozen sweet peas
- Papayas
- Asparagus
- Mangoes
- Eggplant
- Honeydew
- Kiwi
- Cantaloupe
- Cauliflower
- Grapefruit

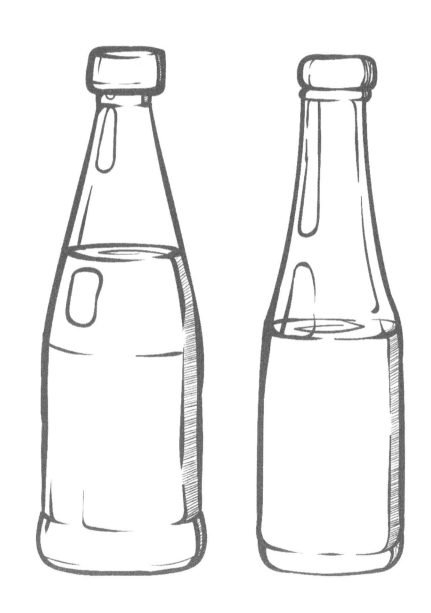

MEASUREMENT CONVERSION TABLES

VOLUME EQUIVALENTS (DRY)

US Standard	Metric (Approx.)
¼ teaspoon	1 ml
½ teaspoon	2 ml
1 teaspoon	5 ml
1 tablespoon	15 ml
¼ cup	59 ml
½ cup	118 ml
1 cup	235 ml

WEIGHT EQUIVALENTS

US Standard	Metric (Approx.)
½ ounce	15 g
1 ounce	30 g
2 ounces	60 g
4 ounces	115 g
8 ounces	225 g
12 ounces	340 g
16 oz or 1 lb	455 g

VOLUME EQUIVALENTS (LIQUID)

US Standard	US Standard (ounces)	Metric (Approx.)
2 tablespoons	1 fl oz	30 ml
¼ cup	2 fl oz	60 ml
½ cup	4 fl oz	120 ml
1 cup	8 fl oz	240 ml
1 ½ cups	12 fl oz	355 ml
2 cups or 1 pint	16 fl oz	475 ml
4 cups or 1 quart	32 fl oz	1 L
1 gallon	128 fl oz	4 L

OVEN TEMPERATURES

Fahrenheit (F)	Celsius (C) (Approx)
250°F	120°C
300°F	150°C
325°F	165°C
350°F	180°C
375°F	190°C
400°F	200°C
425°F	220°C
450°F	230°C

INDEX

Made in the USA
Monee, IL
04 November 2019